SECOND EDITION
SECOND PRINTING 2007

CASH FLOW*

The Practical Art of Earning More From Your Ophthalmology Practice

By John B. Pinto & E. Ann Rose

ASOA

***Selected Readings on Patient Accounts Management, Business Efficiency, Revenue Enhancement, Cost Containment and Durable Profit Improvement**

Prepared under contract to ASOA/ASCRS

ISBN 1-929196-13-X

American Society of Ophthalmic Administrators
an affiliate of American Society of Cataract and Refractive Surgery
4000 Legato Road, Suite 700
Fairfax, Virginia 22033-4033
(703-591-2220)

Contents

This Book is
Dedicated to the Memory of

William E. Rose, Jr.

And to our clients—providers and their staff everywhere—
who improve world eye care each day using the
concepts that Bill helped found.

Pinto's Ten Commandments

1. Hire the best people you can afford. Treat them right.
2. Provide staff with one hour of education for every 79 hours of work.
3. Keep tomorrow's appointment book 100 percent full.
4. Treat every patient as though they were your only customer.
5. Ask every patient to refer a friend.
6. Know your numbers. Cold.
7. Find a surgeon more competent than you, and copy what they do.
8. Sweat every detail. Even the ones that bore you.
9. Financial success is measured in profit per hour, not cases per month.
10. Live on less than 80 percent of your after-tax income. Invest the rest.

About the Authors

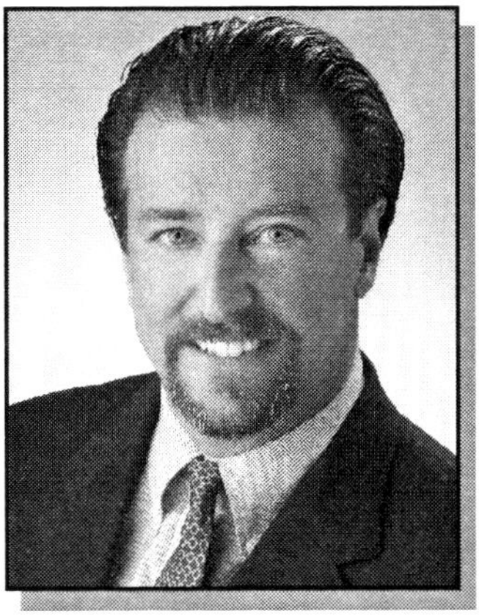

John Pinto is the most-published author in America on ophthalmology practice management topics. He founded J. Pinto & Associates, Inc., an ophthalmic practice management firm, in 1979. Since then, he has provided strategic planning, operations, and marketing advice to pharmaceutical companies, basic science centers, hospitals, multispecialty clinics, and single-specialty facilities. For more than 20 years, a majority of the firm's service has been to ophthalmic practices ranging from small solo practices to high-volume market leaders, teaching centers, and ophthalmic product companies. He is active as a practice consultant in both the U.S. and Europe and has worked and lectured in South America.

Pinto is best known as a strategic planning and economic advisor to practices large and small. In addition to covering most dimensions of modern practice operations management, he is a career advisor, providing individual coaching and contract negotiation services to new graduates and mid-career employed ophthalmologists. As a subspecialty interest, Pinto is very active in refractive surgery and is among the most experienced advisors in the country, helping surgeons with the economic, management, and marketing challenges of this field. His professional life today is rounded out with succession planning, practice appraisals, partner dispute mediation, merger/acquisition counsel, and leadership development for administrators and managing partners.

A prolific writer, Pinto is the author of several books including his classic text, *John Pinto's Little Green Book of Ophthalmology*, along with more recent books, *Turnaround: Twenty-One Weeks to Ophthalmic Practice Survival and Permanent Improvement, Ten Eyecare Practices: Benchmarks for Success*, and *Cash Flow: The Practical Art of Earning More from Your Ophthalmology Practice*, coauthored with E. Anne Rose. Pinto is also the author of *Marketing Your Ophthalmic Practice* (Slack Books, 1987), the first book devoted to the topic. All titles are currently published by the American Society of Ophthalmic Administrators/ASCRS and can be ordered by visiting the ASOA web site www.asoa.org.

Pinto is a member of the editorial boards of *Ocular Surgery News*, *Ophthalmology Management*, and *Comprehensive Ophthalmology*. He is also a regular contributor to numerous other eyecare publications. A new book, *The Women of Ophthalmology*, written with Elizabeth Davis, MD, will be available in 2006.

John Pinto is available for individual practice consulting services to supplement this book. Please contact him at:

J. Pinto & Associates, Inc.
1576 Willow Street
San Diego, CA 92106
(Voice) 619-223-2233
(Fax) 619-223-2253
(E-mail) pintoinc@aol.com
(Web) www.pintoinc.com

A majority of the author's fee associated with this book has been donated to the American Society of Ophthalmic Administrators to further its mission in eyecare management education.

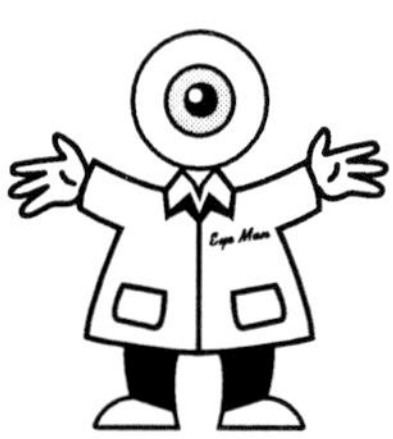

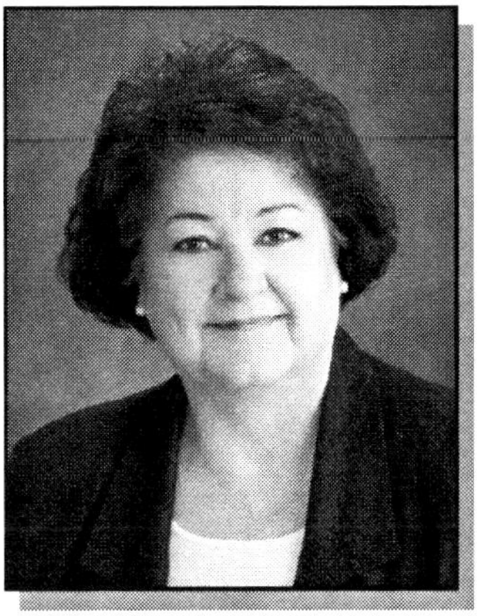

E Ann Rose, owner and president of **Rose & Associates**, is a well-known health care consultant, author, and speaker. In 1980 she and her late husband, William E. (Bill) Rose, formed Rose & Associates, offering a wide variety of Medicare reimbursement and coding services to the ophthalmic community. Her professional experience began in 1966 as a member of the Medicare acquisition team at Blue Cross and Blue Shield of Texas shortly after they were awarded the Medicare claims processing contract. Ann was instrumental in the development of the CMS-1500 claim form. She also served as a team member in developing the paperless claims processing system known today as electronic billing.

In the early 1980's, Ann was heavily involved in the certification of ambulatory surgery centers. She successfully obtained more than 20 Certificates of Need for physicians who were interested in developing surgery centers as part of their medical practice. Using her extensive knowledge of past and current Medicare regulations, Ann now devotes her time and effort to assisting clients with Medicare reimbursement and compliance issues. A few of the services provided by Rose & Associates include, but are not limited to: Extensive on-site chart audits for optimizing reimbursement and maintaining compliance; monthly maintenance programs providing unlimited consultations via phone fax or email; on-site staff training seminars for technicians, coders, physicians or combined training sessions; and assistance with Medicare Fair Hearings and Administrative Law Judge Hearings.

Ann maintains a strong relationship with the American Society of Ophthalmic Administrators (ASOA) and serves as guest speaker at their annual meetings as well as other ophthalmology meetings across the country. She assisted ASOA in editing the Ophthalmic Regulatory Manual (ORM) and provided special coding tips throughout the manual. Ann is on the Board of Advisors for *Ophthalmology Compliance & Reimbursement Insider*, a newsletter devoted to coding, legal, and compliance issues involving ophthalmology and the editorial board of *Ocular Surgery News*. She is also editor and publisher of *The Messenger*, a Rose & Associates coding and reimbursement newsletter written and developed specifically for the specialty of ophthalmology.

For additional information on any of the above services or products, please contact Ann Rose at:

Rose & Associates
402 W. Wheatland, Suite 150
Duncanville, TX 75116-4627
1-800-720-9667
(972) 780-8546 (fax)
E-mail: results@roseandassociates.com

A majority of the authors' fees associated with this book have been donated to the American Society of Ophthalmic Administrators to further their mission in eye care management education.

"When Your outflow exceeds your income,
your updeep becomes your downfall."
James Rohn

Introduction: What is Cash Flow, Anyway?

Mr. Rohn is precisely right. So is the smart-alecky B-school t-shirt that proclaims, "Cash flow is More Important Than Your Mother!"

We would like to apologize in advance to those surgeons and managers who are offended by the use of the word "cash flow" in the context of what remains to us—and likely to you, too—one of the most miraculous and beneficial domains of modern medicine. However, miracles require as much or more money than the mundane, and it falls to us practice advisors to keep the wheels of commerce turning while doctors and their clinical staff get on with the miraculous bits and pieces. Like most people in our position, we cherish the privilege of playing a small part in advancing healthcare for all concerned.

"Cash flow" is the lifeblood, the pulse, of your practice. The formal business definition is that cash flow is the movement of money in and out of your business. It's more than the resultant profit left over at the end of the month. Cash flow is the dynamic, net position emerging from the sum total of your efforts to keep your head above water and the efforts of the environment—payers, competitors, and a few irksome patients—to push your head firmly back under again. The basic difference between positive and negative cash flow can be understood by the average sixth-grader. But the nuances are highly complex. And unfortunately, they don't hand out snorkels in residency training.

Cash flow concepts have only become critical in recent years. More than a decade ago, the typical practice could get by on sketchy annual financial reports. Their financial inflows were stable, and far exceeded their outflows. The greatest practice/business/personal problems revolved around the tax implications of large retained earnings each year.

Looking back panoramically, there have been sweeping changes. Physician payment reform came out of left field. We knew it was eventually coming down the pike, but we didn't know just how it was going to affect the average practice. We thought we would see solo practices go by the wayside.

But they have not faded, although there has been a strong tendency for solo practitioners to take the next difficult hurdle of starting small group practices.

A trend we *do* see is more general practices transitioning to multi-subspecialty clinics. Even die-hard soloists are softening and bringing in part-time subspecialists to augment income and increase patient convenience. Such is progress.

Another, more ominous, trend we see is toward more Medicare auditing. We once saw, among our clients, just an audit or two each year; these were, by and large, fishing expeditions. There was a large concentration in Florida. We now have increased audit traffic from Ohio, New York…the larger states you would expect to see first in an oversight ramp up. The trend has now seemed to proceed nationally. A slated future collapse in the number of regional carriers could like as not increase scrutiny and make auditing efforts more thoroughgoing. More rules, more standards, more care pathway review…more intrusion and more accountability. Some of this is to the good. Carriers are publishing expected standards to help us better understand where the line lies. All the same, under the most literal reading of the fraud and abuse statutes, even innocent errors are severely punishable. Few lily-white, ethical, quality surgeons of our acquaintance are 100 percent error-free. So much is under a potentially dark cloud, especially for high volume doctors, and those whose utilization exceeds peer norms.

Along with these trends, there is a continuing ophthalmic trend toward primary eye care, optical dispensing and bringing optometrists into the practice—not only as paid associates but increasingly as partners. As surgical fees continue to soften, state regulations allow MD-OD partnerships, and the economic rewards for cognitive, non-procedural care grow in importance, we believe this trend will expand.

Almost everything about ophthalmology is more complex than in other specialties. Rather than one or two support staff per doctor, as in other specialties, we have half a dozen or more—sometime significantly more. There are a lot more moving parts. At some levels this would seem to be a disadvantage vis-à-vis the world ahead. But look at it more positively: Ophthalmologists are more experienced than any other specialists at delegating sub-MD care and at using extenders. The potential for passive income to augment falling active income is far more impressive in ophthalmology than in most other specialties.

These higher support staffing levels result in another benefit unique to eye care. We have more people touching the chart and available to cross check for accuracy and completeness. As a result, we think there is the potential for fewer errors and a higher percentage of fees recovered in ophthalmology than in other specialties.

Still, there are common problems in optimizing cash flow in eye care. Most of these problems revolve around sweating the myriad details. Too few practices put sufficient work into maintaining an ongoing relationship with each patient. Recall systems are often spotty or absent. No-show patients are never contacted. Documentation is scant. Over-billing and under-billing is prevalent. Chief complaints and lifestyle impairments are under-charted. Interpretive reports for special testing are absent. Indications for the return appointment are scant or absent. Practices continue to use long-hand, narrative chart notes rather than check-off encounter forms. Assignment of benefit forms is often incomplete.

Even after several years of trying to do things better, the best practices consistently under-bill. They want to "fly under the radar," rather than getting paid a fair fee for services rendered. Because of changing staff, and the lack of written operational procedures, even well-counseled, thoughtful practices can start over and over again each year in getting patient accounts work right.

This isn't due to sloppy work, so much as to over-work and a lack of attention at the top to all of the minor steps that taken together are so meaningful in cash flow terms.

The economic and efficiency "sweet spot" in most of the surgical specialties, ophthalmology and eye care included, is 3-5 principals and a handful of supporting associates. Anything more than this scale can be accompanied by a vexing level of enterprise complexity that can bog down even the most adroit administrator or managing partner. However, there is also a *lower* practice size limit for cash flow efficiency. Anything less than this optimum 3-5 principal scale, and in all but the most profitable small settings it's increasingly impossible to afford the in-house or out-of-house expertise needed to deal with an increasingly complex world. Although pre-paid health care is in moderate retreat, the shear complexity of getting paid for the work that you do in your clinic now exceeds the expertise and systems support of most small, solo practices. A minimum, and likely growing, scale will be needed in the future to simply hang on in the world ahead.

Of course, as profit margins fall, the math of profit enhancement and cost reduction changes drastically. Those reading this who can remember the time when 50 percent profit margins were normal in ophthalmology, can also recall that a 5 percent inefficiency in collections only meant a 10 percent pay cut for the doctors. With the +/- 30 percent margins that are more common today, the same 5 percent inefficiency reduces doctor wages about 17 percent. Ouch!

These complexities are now galloping way, way ahead of the average provider in private practice. None of these complexities is more frustrating—and key to your financial health—than those revolving around the dark art of patient accounts management.

Our original intent was that this book would be a primer for patient accounts management, alone. Like the world, our little project grew in complexity. The present text covers selected topics in patient accounts management. It also covers related themes. Some of the discussion ahead of you in this book is more philosophical in nature. How can doctors and their staff get on the same page regarding practice and profit goals? How does the nature of our relationships with patients and payers directly influence our bottom line? Much of this book has been written to be highly practical, and directly applicable to your practice the next day after you read a given chapter.

In the beginnings, our intent was to co-author this short text. The Rose firm specializes in coding, charting, and reimbursement issues; the Pinto firm covers just about everything with the exception of this, including process engineering for better patient accounts department management. But one-by-one, contributing authors joined the project. We think this has vastly improved the book's value to you. Some of these authors are fellow practice consultants. Others are managers, on the daily front lines in their own practices. We know you'll find their contributions will increase the usefulness this book will have in your own setting.

Optimizing cash flow is obviously not just about revenue management—it's also about cost containment. Ophthalmology is labor intensive, which in recent years has subjected our largest expense to significant "cost-creep." Facility, marketing, and supply costs have similarly ratcheted up. And of course, we have little or no pricing power in ophthalmology, so we are relegated to a defensive posture in many settings.

From our personal perspectives, and we hope yours, too, one of the most important sections of this book is the opening Dedication to William Rose. This is written affectionately by Alan Reider, one of the country's leading health law attorneys and one of ophthalmology's true friends. Bill Rose was one of the founding deans of ophthalmic practice consulting, a pioneer, whose own example of ethical, clear counsel reverberates today in our work with clients. We hope he enjoys looking over our shoulders as this is written, as much as you enjoy reading what lies ahead.

As the second edition of this book goes to press, the U.S. and world economies continue to teeter, a series of drastic Medicare fee cuts looms, and American companies are stepping up efforts to shed employee health care costs. The present era feels very much like the early 1990s, when a soft national economy, the first Gulf War, and burgeoning health costs gave rise to nearly a decade of health care reform experimentation. For ambulatory care providers, including ophthalmologists, these experimental years were not kind. Cataract fees dropped by an average of about a dollar a week. Access to patients, at least for a time, was sharply curtailed in many markets. Apprehension about future changes drove some extremely valuable doctors, vendors, and support staff from the eye care industry.

A decade and more ago, we all thought that electronic medical records and single-payer schemes would all but wipe out the need for care and attention to optimize scheduling, billing, and reimbursement. Instead, we are not really any closer to useful paperless charting, and the demand for attentiveness is twice what was once the case, simply because each dollar billed is so much dearer. The stakes are rising not falling.

We labor with the tyranny of a largely fixed cost business. Unless we experience labor cost deflation, the typical practice will be squeezed between slowly falling fees and slowly rising costs. The next 10 years ahead may be déjà vu all over again. But this time eye care professionals are starting from a much lower productive base, at least in terms of their positive cash flow, and the cash reserves available to weather any difficulty. Like a pilot flying at lower altitudes, errors will be much more punishing.

A kind of "perfect storm" is brewing, with the next decade of health reform, national budget deficits, new dollars allocated to sniffing out so-called "fraud and abuse," and the waxing and waning of elective refractive surgery coinciding with the leading edge of baby boom surgeons retiring just as their investment portfolios continue to bleed. Some few doctors are accelerating their departure from medicine. For others, the only economically and emotionally healthy remedy is to keep polishing their game in the face of a slow (we hope!), incremental, predictable, downward spiral.

The practical economic prognosis is good for many surgeons and their staff:

- Surgeons who can ramp up their scale and become, by slow turns, a little more productive each day
- Doctors who are not afraid to work harder, not only on their clinical skills but their business savvy
- Practices that can diversify their service mix, and not get over-weighted toward one patient type, one payer or one procedure, leaving them more vulnerable to change
- Billing managers who see it as their mission to make sure the team is paid 100 percent appropriately for every single service provided
- Administrators who can stay one step ahead of the next round of managed care reform in their unique markets, and be contractual "haves" rather than "have-nots"

We're hopeful that the material in this book, applied insightfully, appropriately, and vigorously in your own setting, will help you stay ahead of the storm. This is a book meant for doctors and manager alike. Each can make half of the contributions so badly needed to thrive in the years ahead.

Cash Flow

The fact still remains that half of the surgeons, and half of the managers, and half of the practices in America today are performing below average. Which half are you in?

Here's to measurable, gratifying and profitable traction against all apparent trends in the years ahead,

John B. Pinto
J. Pinto & Associates, Inc.
San Diego, California

E. Ann Rose
Rose & Associates
Duncanville, Texas

Dedication to William Rose

By Alan E. Reider

Bill Rose began his career in 1958 working in the Claims and Data Processing Division of Blue Cross/Blue Shield of Mississippi. In 1967 he joined Blue Cross of Louisiana and in 1971 he joined Blue Cross/Blue Shield of Texas. In 1981, after 23 years working with Blue Cross/Blue Shield plans, Bill left to work with physician practices, first as a Vice President of a physician management group and then as Executive Director of a large pathology practice.

But in 1985, Bill Rose had a vision. He saw a need; he saw an opportunity; and he had the courage to take a chance. He established his own consulting firm, providing services to ophthalmology practices. He helped physicians obtain payments they deserved for the work they performed and, perhaps more importantly, he helped them avoid problems.

Bill Rose was ahead of his time. In the mid-1980's, no one had ever heard of a Compliance Program in the healthcare industry. But Bill Rose was bringing ophthalmologists into compliance with the complexities of billing and coding. He limited his work to one specialty because he wanted to be the best that he could be; he wanted to be an expert to one group, not a journeyman to several. And he succeeded. Like EF Hutton, when Bill Rose spoke, ophthalmologists listened.

Perhaps a personal experience best captures the respect that Bill Rose commanded in his field. I met Bill a few years after he began his consulting practice. Soon after we met, we had the opportunity to speak together on a panel. I spoke first and was pleased to see a room full of ophthalmologists, obviously there to hear the insights from the Washington lawyer. Bill's presentation followed. When he was through we received a nice ovation. Shortly after that, Bill and I had a chance to share a panel again. This time, Bill went first. After he finished, I got up, and as soon as I did I watched half of the room empty out. So, I guess the ophthalmologists were not there to hear the words of wisdom from that Washington, D.C. lawyer after all. It was at that point that I made a critical decision — from then on, when Bill and I spoke together, I was going first. I was not going to follow that guy again.

But what made Bill Rose so special? It wasn't just that he was a great speaker. It wasn't just that he was an expert on whom one could rely. It wasn't just that he was an individual whose integrity was impeccable. It wasn't just that when he laughed, the whole room laughed with him. It wasn't just that he was one of those special people with whom you want to be ... when being in his company simply made you feel better. It wasn't just that those of us who knew him because of our work thought of him first as a friend. It was all of those things, and so much more.

Bill Rose was a very special person. He showed us that not only is it possible to achieve the pinnacle of success in your profession, but it is possible also to achieve the pinnacle of success in life, through one's marriage, family, and friends. And Bill Rose did all with style, dignity, and integrity.

Bill Rose has been and will be an inspiration for me. I guess I will have to take back what I said earlier; I hope I am able to follow in his footsteps after all.

Section I: Gushers

Philosophy, Theory, and the Soft Side of Cash Flow Management

"The trouble with the future is that it usually arrives before we are ready for it."

Arnold G. Glasgow

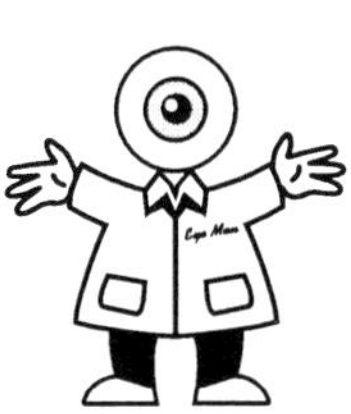

Chapter One: Practice Cash Flow Comes from the Value We Bring to Our Patient Relationships

The scene is an after dinner speech late one night. The consultant is saying to this small group of doctors, "Think of all the remarkable changes coming in healthcare—payment reform, limited access to patients, greater liability exposure, competition, rising costs. Now think of this spiral of changes as a kind of giant corkscrew...and *you're* all, each of you, the cork." Gasps of recognition appeared on every doctor's face.

There are basically two potential responses (institutionally and personally) to this colder, harsher cash flow environment we find ourselves in today. It's an environment that has become so "normal" that it's sometimes hard to remember our professional lives a little more than a decade ago, when the warm glow of new opportunity was evident everywhere. Everywhere.

- You can quietly bite your lip and acquiesce to the changes and accept the fact that each passing year as a surgeon you will have fewer resources to upgrade your skills, your office, your staff and your personal lifestyle. Of course, this will only accelerate the pace at which you slip backward, because acquiescence, once it takes hold, leads to apathy and decline out of all proportion to the environment. Ask wilderness survival instructors and they'll tell you that confidence counts for much more than calories.

OR...

- You can understand that each practice, depending on its location—and more, its gumption—can readily get traction against much of what's slipping backward for the profession right now. There is no better time than now for getting tough and getting going. For taking control. For getting ahead, even in a world where resources slip away.

If you're of the latter impression, and let's do hope that you are, the best place to start is by examining the intersection between two critical words and concepts—the concept of "relationship" and the concept of "value." And most importantly, the compound concept of adding value to your relationships.

These two words are so common, it's easy to overlook their potentially massive impact on the success of your practice. Let's examine this more closely through this practical example. Imagine two doctors, Dr. Success and Dr. Failure. They are each 48 years old, and they practice in the same urban market.

Dr. Success has about 15,000 active patient charts. And he sees these patients on average every 18 months, because he has a sparkling personality—he's the kind of doctor most patients look forward to seeing again for the next visit. His practice has a great recall system, and staff who know how to keep patients from slipping away. Patients are always reminded of their appointments, so the no-show rate is low. Those few lost patients who fail to show up are called immediately and shepherded back into the fold.

Dr. Success is versatile. Although he wasn't subspecialty trained, he's competent, stays current and he's not shy about managing borderline patients that others would typically refer to subspecialists. He also dispenses optical goods, and he has a stake in a local surgery center. As a result, his average revenue yield per patient visit is $185. Because he stays healthy, Dr. Success is energetic, and can see about 55 patients a day with energy to spare. In fact, he's so energetic, and so loves his work, that he only takes three weeks off a year. He operates one day a week and has four full days of clinic.

So as you can see, Dr. Success has it all in the relationship and value departments. He has lots of relationships, these relationships are well cemented, and he exchanges a lot of value for a lot of income. His practice revenue is high—about $1.9 million a year. Dr. Success believes in sharing his success, so he pays his competent staff well, their motivation is high, and they help to perpetuate his success. Even so, Dr. Success has a 40 percent profit margin, and has a pre-tax income of about $760,000 a year, more than twice the national averages.

By contrast, Dr. Failure, who has been in practice just as long as Dr. Success, has only about 7,000 active patient charts, because he's not very good at developing and maintaining relationships. Dr. Failure sees each patient on average only about once every 24 months. His personality is anything but sparkling. In fact, although he was originally trained as well as Dr. Success, Dr. Failure comes across as uncertain when speaking to patients—and this uncertainty is perceived as disinterest, or worse, incompetence.

His practice recall system is almost non-existent. Dr. Failure figures if a patient isn't smart enough to remember to come back in 1 or 2 years, there's no point nagging them...they deserve to get lost. Patients are sometimes reminded of their appointments, but the charts of patients who fail to show up are put right back in the stacks. Dr. Failure loves medical meetings because they're such a great break from the drudgery and stress of practice. But Dr. Failure rarely attends lectures or even networks with his peers. He figures that with his hard job he deserves to sleep in once in a while, hang by the pool, and go shopping.

Dr. Failure may be a little lazy, but at least he's clinically ethical. As his professional skills have eroded year-by-year, he's freely delegated subspecialty care that was increasingly beyond his grasp. He doesn't dispense glasses, and he's never been invited to be a surgery center partner because his case volumes are simply too low. As result of all this, Dr. Failure's average revenue yield per patient visit is only $135. Dr. Failure is somewhat less than energetic, as you can gather. So he runs out of gas whenever he has to see more than 30 patients a day, although his average is about 25. Any more than a couple of work-in patients leave him glaring at his beleaguered appointment clerk.

He works just four days a week, and he doesn't even come back to the office after his handful of surgical cases on Wednesday. The combination of not particularly enjoying his practice, and being so exhausted by it, means that Dr. Failure takes eight weeks off a year, sometimes more.

As you can see, Dr. Failure is in real trouble. He has relatively few patient relationships after all these years in practice, these relationships are poor, and he exchanges small value for small recompense. His practice revenue is only about $450,000 a year. Dr. Failure can barely afford his own salary, much less his staff, so he keeps a low-paid, over-taxed skeleton crew, which reinforces their poor interaction with patients. By keeping other costs trimmed, Dr. Failure ekes out a 35 percent profit margin and has a pre-tax income of about $158,000 a year, or roughly 70 percent of the national average, and just about a fifth of Dr. Success' income.

There are hundreds of ways to establish and maintain more and better patient relationships, and hundreds more ways of adding value. Hundreds of ways to become a "Dr. Success." Sometimes it's hard to see this abstractly by thinking all at once about the multitude of patients that you serve. Think, instead, about just a single, typical patient, "Ms. Davis." Someone you saw yesterday. And ask yourself:

- Did Ms. Davis have a uniformly pleasant experience when she set up her first appointment? Did she receive a followup note welcoming her to the practice and telling her about the practice's policies and scope of services?

- Was the patient or colleague who referred Ms. Davis to your care properly thanked for their referral?
- Did you call Ms. Davis in advance of her appointment? Did you ask her if she had any questions about directions, bringing her medications, or allowing enough time for a complete exam?
- Did the front desk treat Ms. Davis like an old, returning friend? Or did they treat her like an inconvenience, another number to process?
- Was she helped patiently with any paperwork and seen within 20 minutes of her appointment time?
- Did the tech who started Ms. Davis' exam march many steps ahead while escorting her down the hall to Room Two, or did she walk by her side, aiding her if necessary and enjoying a moment of small talk?
- Did staff refer to Ms. Davis by her proper name unless she insisted otherwise?
- Did you really address Ms. Davis' chief complaint, or gloss over this to get to the cataract surgery that you thought was most important?
- Did you look Ms. Davis directly in the eye (and not just with your slit lamp) when you spoke to her about her chief complaint? Did you touch her reassuringly? Compliment her on her sharp mind or snappy attire?
- Was Ms. Davis told, "A little stick here" or similar words before her injection, or did you just jab her without warning?
- If she was brave, or even if she wasn't, did you tell her, "Good job?"
- Does Ms. Davis understand what comes next in her treatment plan?
- Does she understand the importance of keeping her next appointment?
- Was Ms. Davis gently and appropriately exposed to other services that you provide? Or did you just assume from appearances she was on a fixed income and could never afford new glasses or botox injections?
- Did you ask Ms. Davis to be sure to refer her friends to the practice? Did you give her cards or brochures to make this easier to do?
- Were her charges explained at checkout? Was a tech tracked down to help answer any last-minute questions?
- Did someone at the checkout desk wish her good day by name? Were they at least the 3rd or 4th person to thank her for coming in that day?
- If Ms. Davis was given a test that will require subsequent interpretation and report writing, will you keep her in the loop promptly on her results?
- If she was a particularly worried patient, will Ms. Davis get a reassuring call from your staff in a few days just to check to see how things are going?

- If she bought glasses, will she get a call in a few weeks to see if they're still comfortable or need adjusting?

Finally, by the end of her exam, was Ms. Davis's relationship with you—and yours with her—stronger than when you started? Perfect! That's the surest measure of value exchanged.

Will it get harder and harder to do all of this in the future? The answer is an emphatic yes. Patient expectations are rising just as your resources—and especially the emotional resources needed to be so *darned* nice for so *much less reimbursement* at every encounter—are diminishing. But fortunately, most of the attributes needed to improve the value exchange in a service relationship don't cost a dime. Your same staff who are surly to patients now can learn to be sweet for free if you provide a positive role model and reinforcement, accompanied by stiff consequences for continued poor patient service.

None of us involved in this wonderful profession of eye care—whether we're surgeons or surgical supporters—like change. But we have to learn how to ride down the road in alignment with the way the traffic is flowing or risk getting run over. Our most worthy competitors are certainly going with the flow and sharpening their relationships...increasing the value they convey to patients at every visit. Their cash flow will show the results. Don't be like Herman in the small story we'll end this with...

> *...Senior citizen, Herman, was driving down the freeway. His car phone rang. "Herman, Herman! Are you OK?!?" says Herman's wife through the phone with a sound of concern. "Of course, Millie," Herman says. "Thank goodness," his wife replies. I was just listening to the news on the radio. There's a car going the wrong way on the interstate." "It's worse than that," Herman replies. "It's not just one car, it's hundreds of them!!"*

Chapter Two: Sharing Common Goals from the Boardroom to the Break Room

By Stephen W. Gilkeson

In an era of declining third-party reimbursement and increasing operating expense, modern medical practices must continually seek new ways to maintain acceptable profit margins. While these efforts might include cutting back on services to reduce expenses or expansion into new service offerings to increase revenues, for our practice increased profitability has resulted from increasing the productivity of the current practice structure.

As physician owners and business managers, we shoulder the final responsibility for the financial successes of our individual practices. We also understand, or at least we should understand, the cash flow implications our decisions can have on the bottom line. But what about empowering those assets that are central to the implementation of our strategic policies, namely our employees?

Over the years, our practice has found that when we set in place a strategic plan for our entire organization, it is imperative for success that we define each individual employee's contribution to those goals and provide them with the tools for success. Working both as an individual and as a group within the practice, staff members must understand their impact upon bottom line performance.

While there are several factors at play in this, it has been our experience that increases in staff productivity have provided the greatest results in meeting the bottom line performance goals of our practice. We call this ongoing process "moving management from the boardroom to the break room." The following pearls flow from how we've put this slogan into action.

The Mission Statement

When an employee begins work with our practice, we try to instill a sense of teamwork right from the beginning. One of our most important tools in this process is the mission statement.

As with most projects within our practice, this statement was designed through a group effort, and was developed during a series of meetings to identify our practice strengths and the goals we wished to achieve. The following are highlights from that statement:

- We strive to do things right and to do the right things;

- We strive to provide our customers with the best quality eye care;

- We will provide vision care services in a professional manner with a personal touch;

- By treating our patients like friends and family, we will insure that they experience exceptional customer service at each and every visit to the Young Eye Institute;

- We will provide our customers with dependable, quality workmanship;

- We will continually focus on the future – educating ourselves on new technology and techniques that will benefit our patients;

- As individuals, we will be ambassadors of the Young Eye Institute in professional as well as personal situations; and

- We will be successful in achieving our goals by working together as a team.

Having a clear, well-defined statement of objectives provides our staff with the overall goals of our organization from the moment they begin their employment.

In addition, by displaying this statement in our reception area, it allows our patients to judge us daily on our performance in meeting these goals.

Empowering Your Staff

Without providing tools for your staff to reach the goals of the practice, all the policies in the world mean nothing. That is why, over the years, we've refined a program in which every member of our team shares in the success of our practice. It's a concept we refer to as "PEP," and it involves addressing three important criteria:

- Patient Satisfaction
- Expense Reduction
- Productivity Increase

Patient Satisfaction

In the early years, we invested a sizeable amount of our marketing budget in external promotion to build brand awareness. But, as our practice has grown and matured, we've focused more of our energies and finances on internal forms of marketing and promotion.

Our entire staff is very attuned to maintaining and improving levels of patient satisfaction throughout our practice. They know that the strongest referral source is from one patient to another, and how vital these types of referrals are to the health of our practice. That is why no detail in patient care is too small, and every recommendation to our staff from a patient is given careful consideration by management during weekly meetings.

In addition, we conduct regular patient satisfaction surveys to determine what we're doing right and where we can improve our service. What you can measure, you can manage, and by providing feedback to staff from our patients, we can actually see the fruits of our labor. We share these results with our staff, both the good and the bad, to build stronger relations with the patients we serve.

As a result of these efforts, over the last 5 years we've been able to reduce external marketing expenses by well over 50 percent while maintaining a very healthy rate of growth. Word-of-mouth referrals now represent over 60 percent of total patient referrals and it continues to grow. Again, by sharing these statistics with our staff, we are able to prove that by doing the right things and doing them right, the entire organization benefits.

Expense Reduction

This represents the second area we focus on in the PEP program. As a group, we work diligently to cut the fat within our practice without touching the muscle.

Without the participation of your entire staff in expense reduction, it's nearly impossible to make any headway in this area. First of all, without having the systems in place to measure expenses on regular basis, it's hard to determine what is fat and what isn't fat within the practice. Secondly, without feedback from the staff members who will be affected, your efforts may be undermined through lack of implementation.

To augment our success, we hold regular monthly meetings with clinical and surgical departments to review cost saving measures. In these meetings, we try to communicate to all staff members the importance of reducing waste and the impact reductions can have upon our bottom line performance. We also openly solicit suggestions from individual staff members, and reward those employees with the best recommendations. After all, they're on the front lines, and often provide us with the best ideas for cost savings.

For example, it's not uncommon for utility rates in our area to rise four to six percent every year. For a facility as large as ours, this would represent a significant increase in overhead if left unchecked. By sharing information on utility costs with our employees, they better understand the importance of conserving energy in ways as simple as making sure the programmable thermostats are operating in "away" mode when the building is vacant over weekends and holidays.

Telephone usage is another major concern within our practice. That is why we use software to monitor incoming and outgoing line usage, and present this data in our monthly management meetings. Through visual example, we are able to show our staff how important it is to keep our phone lines open so that patients can reach us to schedule appointments. In turn, this also cuts down on the time our receptionists spend answering personal phone calls for other employees, as well as the number of incoming phone lines needed to handle call loads.

Perhaps the greatest strides we've made in expense reduction have been in the area of paperwork reduction. Our staff has made a major push to reduce the number of "trees we cut down" each year through computerization.

Three years ago, our practice established an "intranet" on our computer server, whereby financials, customer surveys and office policy and procedure manuals are placed online within our office. Since most of our employees have access to secure terminals, information is now at their fingertips, and not stored in some bulky notebook or multiple policy manuals.

Just as important is the fact that the information contained within our intranet is "real time," meaning data is seconds or minutes old instead of weeks or months old. Not only does this allow our staff greater flexibility in our decision making process as practice dynamics change, but it also reduces the voluminous amounts of physical space necessary for record storage.

Productivity Increase

In a service organization such as healthcare, asset productivity is the lifeblood of favorable cash flow. As such, this area holds the greatest promise in meeting the strategic goals of our practice.

While staff are your practice's most valuable resource by far, their associated costs are ordinarily the largest practice expense. Therefore, the greater productivity we can derive from each staff member, the greater the impact on the overall bottom-line performance of the organization.

As I mentioned in the beginning, all staff members must be aware of the individual and group related impact upon reaching the strategic goals of the practice. This can be accomplished by providing each staff member with a detailed job description, and transferring to that individual performance accountability for their position and their department.

For example, in our practice we make extensive use of videotapes while conducting time/motion studies of our staff duties. By shaving seconds/minutes off a patient's visit, we are able to provide our customers with more efficient service. This also allows us to utilize our human resource and physical assets to their fullest potential.

In our medical clinic we can tape entire check-in procedures for different patient visits, and review these minute-by-minute to reduce patient flow bottlenecks. We then combine our findings with our computerized patient schedule, and determine optimal times for procedures such as special testing to increase room turnover.

Taping also works well to increase the productivity of our surgery center. As a group, the surgeon and the surgeon's staff are able to plan every move made during a patient's surgical procedure, thereby improving bottom line efficiency and facility revenues.

Finally, videotaping also serves as a tool for improving training of our new employees. Our office maintains a large training library designed to get new staff members up and running with the least amount of downtime to our other, more experienced staff members. In addition, if a new procedure is added to our clinic or surgery center, we can conduct concise instruction in a group setting.

Automated testing has also played an important role in improving staff productivity within our practice. By having a good grasp of scheduling, patient flow and practice financial data, we know when the opportunity presents itself for the automation of a particular procedure. Not only does this allow us to see more patients, but many times it reduces our need to hire additional full-time equivalents to meet patient demand.

Bringing it all Together

Expanding management from the boardroom to the break room really hasn't taken a huge effort to positively impact the bottom line success of our practice. It has broadened the base of fiscal responsibility and galvanized the partnership between upper management and staff members to reach a set of common goals.

To quote Oliver Wendell Holmes, "The mind, once expanded to the dimensions of larger ideas, never returns to its original size." By empowering our employees with knowledge, giving them the tools to reach common goals and providing them with feedback on a daily basis, we are well on our way to prospering in today's challenging economy.

Chapter Three: Compliance and Positive Cash Flow Can Exist in Harmony

By Alan E. Reider

Despite the impression of many physicians and other health care providers, "compliance" and "compliance plans" are not synonymous with decreased revenue and unbearable practice overhead costs. In fact, compliance with all applicable federal or state laws and health care program/plan requirements could save money for a practice and may even result in increased revenue. While there is no magic formula or absolute means of protection from the inherent risks of operating within the increasingly complex health care payment systems, a well-designed and conscientiously implemented compliance program can provide a physician practice with the tools necessary to meet its business objectives and operate in an ethical and legal manner.

All health care providers who treat beneficiaries of the federal health care programs are expected to furnish their services in a manner consistent with the rules and regulations governing the programs and to ensure that their claims submitted to the government are true and accurate. A compliance program is a series of internal policies and procedures voluntarily undertaken by health care providers that are designed to assist them in meeting both of these goals through the prevention, detection, and resolution of conduct that does not conform to a practice's ethical and business goals. Compliance programs may be tailored to deal with any number of specific practice operations, regulatory requirements and business relationships. Each program, however, should cover the four principal compliance risk areas for physician practices identified by the Office of the Inspector General (OIG) of the Department of Health and Human Services (HHS), i.e., (1) coding and billing, (2) reasonable and necessary services, (3) documentation, and (4) improper inducements, kickbacks, and self-referrals.

I. The Benefits and Costs of Compliance Programs

A. Benefits

The potential benefits of having an effective compliance program are both financial and legal in nature. An effective program can increase an entity's cash flow by: Improving the efficiency and accuracy of a practice's coding and billing systems; identifying physicians that consistently downcode their services or fail to bill for services (likely out of fear they might receive an inappropriate payment from the government), and then, educating them to ensure that they understand how to bill for all services for which payment is rightfully due; isolating billing errors, thereby enabling the practice to resubmit claims more quickly; and improving documentation to reduce the possibility that claims are denied.

Compliance programs also help protect practices' revenue by preventing improper business dealings and the attendant liabilities that could prove costly, even financially devastating. Although continuous compliance monitoring cannot assure that errors will not be made nor can it eliminate the potential for liability, it can decrease the possibility that a practice will engage in conduct that the government may challenge as abusive. Without doubt, the legal and expert consultant fees associated with defending against allegations made by the government would far exceed those spent in implementing a compliance plan.

Compliance programs also have the potential to reduce financial exposure for practices in situations where the government concludes that a practice has billed improperly or engaged in otherwise improper conduct. The government has acknowledged that a practice that has an effective compliance program in place creates an inference of good faith and, as a result, the government likely will adopt a much less aggressive enforcement position. In fact, the OIG has stated that the single most influential factor in its decision as to what penalty, if any, to impose on a provider that has engaged in conduct which violates applicable rules or regulations is whether the provider has made a legitimate attempt to prevent improper conduct through implementation of an effective compliance program. Depending on the type of allegation made against a practice, this protection could be the difference between the practice being required to make a simple refund of an overpayment or paying an extraordinary sum of money. Indeed, violations of the Federal Civil False Claims Act, the government's primary legal tool against billing improprieties, are subject to damages of three times the amount paid on a claim plus a penalty of between $5,500 and $11,000 per claim. Thus, a practice found to have submitted 100 false claims for which it was paid $50 per claim (or a total of $5,000) could be liable to the government for between $565,000 and $1,115,000.

Threats of False Claims Act prosecution should not be taken lightly. Several years ago approximately 10 large ophthalmology practices settled FCA allegations made by the government that the billing company hired by the practice, Income Rx, had filed inappropriate claims on behalf of the practices. While Income Rx was indicted and eventually pled to a criminal charge, each of the practices was forced to settle for a multiple of up to three times the amount they had been paid by Medicare. In some cases, the repayment exceeded $2 million.

B. Costs

The benefits of a compliance program are not realized without some investment of time and money. Nevertheless, when asked, providers who have implemented compliance programs generally state that the actual and potential benefits of having a compliance program exceed the expense of implementing and maintaining the program.

The cost of a program should be considered in two parts: The expenses related to the initial development and launch of the program and the expenses required to maintain it on a day-to-day basis. Ultimately, the cost of a compliance program will be driven by the size of the practice and the number and complexity of any business arrangements to which the practice and/or its physician-members are a party. Other factors include the level of compliance at which the practice is functioning at the time the program is implemented and the degree to which a practice already has compliance expertise in-house from which to draw.

As part of the initial development of a compliance program, practices are encouraged to undergo a thorough "baseline audit," i.e., a legal and coding review of all of the practice's principal operations. This audit, which is recommended by the AMA and OIG in their compliance plan guidance, is generally the most expensive portion of the program but may be the most critical. To the extent possible, a practice should begin a compliance program with the knowledge that it has taken all reasonable steps to put its operations in order.

The baseline audit is a review of the structure of the practice, all relevant contracts and other relationships with suppliers and referral sources, the practice's administration and patient relations, the accuracy of the practice's billing and coding systems and medical record documentation. The purpose of this baseline audit is three-fold. First, the audit provides an objective assessment of the practice's compliance in areas considered to be high risk in order to identify problems that require attention before the compliance program is implemented. Second, the audit highlights other areas of concern that will require behavioral or systems changes and a period of time in order for the practice to improve. Third, the audit services as the foundation for the practice to establish performance goals which the practice will strive to achieve. Examples of performance goals vary from achieving a lower disallowance rate in internal audits to amending a practice's charge slip format to assure more accuracy in billing and coding.

On average, the cost of the baseline audit for a small practice with limited business relationships other than employment of a small office staff and possible leasing office space and/or equipment, generally is in the $10,000-$15,000 range. On the other hand, the cost for a larger practice that is involved in more complex business arrangements such as joint ventures with referral sources, or the ownership and operation of a free-standing diagnostic testing facility, may be as much as $40,000.

The cost of developing the compliance program documents, and developing and performing the initial education and training program, depends on the extent to which the practice uses its own resources or contracts with consultants or lawyers to provide assistance. Depending on the practice's choice, the cost for this phase could range from $2,000 to more than $10,000, again, depending on the size of the practice and the work required.

Finally, the expenses incurred annually to maintain the compliance functions generally are far less than those associated with implementation and are related largely to the cost related to the additional duties of the compliance officer and regular auditing and monitoring.

C. Resistance to Compliance Programs

So, WHY, despite the potential financial benefits and legal protections offered by compliance programs, do many practices and physicians continue to ignore compliance? Aside from cost, a frequently cited reason is fear that the compliance effort may uncover problems that may lead to action by the government. This concern, however, reflects a fundamental misunderstanding about the purpose and effect of compliance programs.

There should be no question that if, through a compliance review, a practice discovers that it has been paid inappropriately, it must refund that amount to Medicare or the applicable payor. Notwithstanding this obligation, the OIG has made it clear in its Model Compliance Plan for Physician Practices ("Model Plan"), that under the law, physicians and other health care providers are not subject to criminal or civil penalties for honest mistakes, errors, or even simple negligence. For example, the False Claims Act applies only to prohibited conduct undertaken with actual knowledge, reckless disregard, or deliberate ignorance of the falsity of the claim submitted to the government. Therefore, in order for the government or a whistleblower to prove an FCA violation, it must show either that the provider knew that a claim was false when it was submitted to the government, or that it was purposely negligent. Consequently, it would be difficult for the government to demonstrate that a practice was reckless or purposefully negligent in circumstances where an effective compliance plan was in place, and the problem was discovered by the practice. If, on the other hand, the government discovers the problem, it would be far more difficult for the provider to argue the error was an honest mistake, particularly if the practice did not have a compliance program in place.

The need for compliance programs is not limited to those practices that serve Medicare or other government program beneficiaries. Most states have laws that mirror the federal fraud and abuse laws. Those laws impose similar obligations on physicians regardless of whether a private payor (including the patient) or federal payor is involved. In some cases, state laws may be broader in scope and carry more severe penalties. Thus, compliance applies to all practices, regardless of the patient or payor mix.

II. Implementing and Documenting an Effective Compliance Program

A. Establishing Effectiveness

In order to realize the benefits of a compliance program — both with respect to the financial and operational improvements as well as the legal protections it may provide — the program must be "effective." While effectiveness is not a specifically defined term, it does not mean that a compliance program is expected to identify and resolve every possible payment or regulatory problem, but it does require a practice to make a good faith attempt to do so. Furthermore, certain fundamental elements must be put into place and must function effectively. Specifically, to demonstrate effectiveness, a compliance program must include the following seven basic components:

- Implementation of compliance and practice policies and procedures through the development of written standards (often referred to as the Standards of Conduct);
- Designation of a compliance officer who is delegated sufficient authority to oversee the ongoing compliance efforts and to enforce practice standards;
- Execution of a regular and appropriate module of training;
- Development of a system of internal monitoring;

- Establishment of a system to respond and correct compliance violations;
- Cultivation of an environment of open communication; and
- Installation of a disciplinary process that is applied when appropriate.

The degree to which these components function as anticipated generally is measured against the performance goals set by the practice based on the results of its baseline audit, as discussed in the previous section. Thus, documentation that performance goals have been met is some evidence of an effective compliance program. The OIG has acknowledged a number of other indicators to determine whether a program likely is effective. These indicators include sufficient funding of a practice's compliance efforts, participation by an entity's medical staff in all aspects of the compliance program, including training, auditing and serving on the compliance committee, receptiveness and responsiveness to all good faith reports of possible compliance issues, documented instances of refunding overpayments to all payers including patients, and routine auditing of medical records and claims. To be an effective compliance plan, a practice cannot simply develop the necessary documentation and put it on the shelf.

B. A Few Specifics

An effective compliance program must be a dynamic and ongoing process and contain each of the seven components listed above. While each component serves an important function, the OIG has acknowledged that the significance of the various components to a specific practice's compliance program will vary depending on the size and culture of the practice. The OIG also has pointed out that it expects that training and auditing to be critical to all programs.

i. Training

A well-designed and interesting training protocol is a critical first step in securing employees' commitment to a compliance program. Training is mandatory and should: Educate the practice personnel, including all medical and clinical staff, about the practice's compliance mission; insure that the employees understand that they have an explicit obligation to report any suspected violations of the Standards of Conduct; and instill the philosophy that compliance takes team work across all departments.

There is considerable overlap in the responsibilities delegated to human resources personnel and to employees handling compliance, particularly in the areas of training as well as discipline and complaint follow-up. Experienced compliance officers report that many of the initial reports received through compliance program reporting systems and hotlines relate to employment and labor issues. Thus, practices should consider training the individuals in these roles to anticipate the nature of issues likely to be raised.

ii. Auditing and Monitoring

As emphasized above, every compliance program must provide for periodic internal audits of the practice's operations. Internal audits may be divided into two categories: Those aimed at certain routine operations such as documentation and billing; and those aimed at investigating reports of possible inappropriate conduct. The OIG Model Plan recommends that periodic audits of the compliance program be conducted at least once a year. Depending on the expertise required for the nature of the issue under review, the audit team may consist of employees, an outside billing consultant, an attorney, an accountant or a combination of the above. In all cases, the compliance officer should oversee the design and mechanics of the audit.

A practice also should have a mechanism to assure that all parts of its program, such as compliance with its training protocol and consistency in disciplinary actions, are maintained appropriately. Further, annual employee surveys and exit interviews can be very useful methods to compile informative feedback about a program and compliance matters generally. All employees that terminate their relationships with a practice should be questioned regarding any possible compliance violations they believe exist at the practice. They should also be encouraged to provide constructive input on how to improve the compliance program.

C. A Final Note: Outsourcing Compliance Efforts

Except for the development and adoption of the Standards of Conduct, much, if not all, of the day-to-day tasks of a running an effective compliance program may be outsourced to external compliance consultants. Outsourcing is a very important option for smaller practices, as it enables those without any significant internal compliance experience to bring expert capability to its program.

Health care fraud enforcement activity by both the federal and state governments continues to grow. Each year new health care practices come under fire, leaving physicians constantly trying to ensure they are not the next targets, while still running successful practices. The rules do not prohibit physicians from optimizing their reimbursement provided their efforts to do so stay within the boundaries of the law. Compliance plans help physicians identify these boundaries and to succeed within them.

Chapter Four:
Positioning Your Practice Toward the Most Profitable Sectors of Eye Care

More than any other specialty, ophthalmology has an amazingly broad diversity of subspecialty, elective, and retail services and products to provide to patients. Some of these services and products are more enjoyable or professionally rewarding. Some of these are more financially rewarding. Some have a high barrier to entry and require substantial education or capital. And some take almost no time, effort, risk or capital to offer to your patients.

Most readers have probably arrived in their present practice settings through a series of well-placed accidents. Few optometrists or surgeons make a string of conscious decisions about their professional destinies, which can lead to a lot of latter-day regrets and jealousies.

All but the most satisfied optometrists express the private question, "Would it have really been that much harder to go to medical school?" Pediatric ophthalmologists will commonly report that they adore their patients and their professional challenges but feel unfairly treated economically. Academic and HMO surgeons frequently express regrets that they didn't beat a path to private practice—they look enviously at the independence and superior earnings of their freelancing colleagues in the community. These independent general ophthalmologists, in turn, look at their higher-volume refractive surgery or retinal surgery colleagues and wish that they could also enjoy million-dollar-plus wages. Perched at the top of the ophthalmic food chain, retinologists envy few of their generalist colleagues (but they can have a mildly green streak when it comes to comparing notes with their Wall Street zillionaire neighbors down the street!)

Each of these professionals in the spectrum of eye care has a choice. No, it's probably not practical for most pediatric ophthalmologists to drop everything and train as a retinal surgeon. But everyone can look at the range of services and products they're selling to their patients today and ask, "Is my mix right? Am I balanced correctly between surgical and medical care? Should I add dispensing, or eliminate an unproductive satellite office?"

One of the most common balancing questions on the table for a great number of surgeons today is the proper balance between performing refractive surgery and tending to general/geriatric eye care in your practice.

Since the early 1980's, when vision correction surgery first arose as a commercially viable subspecialty in America, surgeons have considered the option of focusing all or nearly all of their career attentions on RK, PRK, LASIK and derivative procedures. In the last 20 years we've now had a chance to see numerous refractive surgery volume downturns, as these procedures have fallen in and out of favor with the buying public and as consumer discretionary dollars have changed with the general economic climate.

However, as happens at the end of every boom cycle, some refractive surgeons are always left a little too unbalanced toward refractive surgery and a little too estranged from the bread and butter of their general practice.

This time around, as in circa 1990/1991, unfortunate refractive surgery bias decisions—and the consequences of these decisions—started emerging in early 2001 as the economy softened. Any surgeon with more than about a third of their income derived from Lasik surgery started to experience a steep profit decline, which continues as this book goes to press. The hallmarks of this kind of unbalance include:

- Geriatric and general marketing budgets have been emptied out to pay for LASIK promotion. Each month the cost-per-lead keeps rising, and the conversion rate from consultation to surgery decreases;

- Recall systems have fallen flat, because staff and doctors got in the habit of thinking of patients as a short-term surgical fee "pop" rather than a slow, long-term annuity "sizzle;"

- The purchase of soon-obsolesced, expensive excimer equipment and keratomes have created high fixed overhead and have tied up capital and borrowing power that might be crucial to make it through the LASIK doldrums (or be able to profitably serve a future lower-reimbursing patient base.);

- Fortunes have been spent furnishing lavish, "Keep up with the Dr. Joneses" clinical facilities. Such facilities may be necessary for young, elective surgical patients but can leave senior patients a little overwhelmed and thinking, "So *this* is why my doctor needs a $30 refraction fee;"

- Practices that converted to LASIK-only patients have lost the "institutional memory" for how to correctly bill and get paid by complex third-party payment systems. Indeed, a few now-faltering LASIK practices, without any convention al claims-submission software, are having to start over from scratch to be able to simply bill Medicare; and

- Local competitors have taken advantage of your LASIK practice's niche focus to develop stronger ties not only with the senior public but also with important referral sources. It could take years in some cases for you to catch up.

Restoring a Balance

For a moment, think of your practice as a composite of many smaller companies. You have the "LASIK Company," the "Cataract Company," and the "Glaucoma Company." And perhaps even the "Dry Eye Company." The list is—and should be—rather long. Each of these practice segments clamor for attention, for resources. They demand capital for specialized equipment. They demand your time to stay current and to orient staff. Each demands your focus. You should conduct every patient encounter with ALL of your services in mind.

Ask yourself, without being overly predatory, "Did I provide every patient I saw this past week with the full array of services they need and that we're in a position to provide? Or was I so focused on finding my next LASIK candidate that I walked right past several opportunities to better serve the patients I do have in abundance? Your honest answer to these questions will not only make you a better physician but a better business person. This will help cash flow immensely.

We see this all the time during practice site visits, and you can see the same thing in your own practice. Pull a few charts at random. Examine them to see what additional services could have been provided to each patient. Common gaps include dry eye treatment, a recall order that was not charted properly, and glasses that were never ordered because the doctor didn't talk about the practice's optical. At the same time, you should look to see if the charted services are shown in your computer system, and if they were paid. It's not at all unusual, even with a desultory scanning of the chart, to find all kinds of dollars that have fallen through the cracks in the rush of the clinic day.

It may not seem like much of a contribution, but in the typical practice setting, if you can just sell another $15-$20 worth of appropriate services to the average patient, you can give yourself a six-figure pay raise. Of course, this math works in a similarly leveraged fashion in reverse, when payers reduce the allowable fee. In such cases, you should expect to see your income slingshot south.

Getting back to a greater focus on the general and geriatric eye care sectors and away from any sectors like LASIK or elective plastics than have been hurt recently, obviously takes more than just having your head back in the game. It takes specific, focused, and sometimes costly action.

One core tactical action is going to be shifting your marketing and advertising budget. The best generic advice, applicable to most settings, is that the LASIK media and marketing budget should be pulled back 40 percent, while pushing half or more of this back into geriatric and general eye care promotion. Most active LASIK surgeons have already gotten comfortable with relatively high media budgets; all they need to do is shift audience and market segments. In re-positioning your practice, you can quickly pass your more timid competitors. This is especially the case if you employ some of the patient service enhancements discussed in Chapters One and Two.

How should you get your old patient base back? Patient-to-patient referral still works best. But if your base of seniors has tapered, you need to reintroduce yourself to the marketplace. That doesn't have to be expensive, at least compared to LASIK advertising. *And it's far easier to get back into cataracts than it is to start refractive surgery.*

More good news, of course, is that unlike the typical LASIK patient, your senior patient will likely receive services for years. Inasmuch as cognitive and dispensing revenue are growing at a faster pace than surgical fees, and certainly faster than LASIK fees, the global revenue and profit yield per new senior patient is far higher than for the one-time younger patient.

Here are additional check-offs for re-balancing a general practice that has strayed too far into refractive surgery:

- General practice marketing costs should run about 3 percent to 5 percent of the revenue from that part of your practice, year in and year out; 8-15 percent is necessary for the LASIK portion of your practice;
- Make sure a live operator picks up your phone during all business hours;
- Get back into health fairs, senior nutrition site screenings, OD outreach and other traditional general eye care marketing tactics—you'll be amazed how many of these niches have been abandoned in recent years;
- If you got into LASIK because you were bored with cataracts, find some new, leading-edge aspect of cataract surgery that's interesting. Come to think of it, cataract surgery ***IS*** refractive surgery, isn't it?

- Adopt a zero-defects recall system and polish customer service. A great geriatric eye care advertising program can potentially make wobbly operations fail faster; and
- Aim to build your total cataract case volumes to 60 or more cases a month, alone or in concert with compatible partners or associates, so you can eventually add a surgical facility. Most regulatory hurdles to ASC development have been falling for years now; ancillary facility income is critical to replace cataract professional fee income. However, there is no certainty that facility fees will continue to rise as they have of late.

Remember that eye care is a largely fixed-cost service business. A 10 percent drop in revenue typically can result in a 20+ percent drop in profits. Sustaining revenue is critical. If you can't sustain revenue by re-positioning the practice, you must reduce operating costs.

A discussion of repositioning and re-balancing your practice begs the larger topic of how you're managing your entire financial life, including retirement planning. For many surgeons, a poor business climate can have more effect on your long-term retirement plans than on your near-term lifestyle. Not only is your income dropping, but your investment portfolio may be as well. Surprisingly few surgeons understand how close or far they are from financial independence. Now is the time to know where you realistically stand. While there's no substitute for a face-to-face expert, such as an accountant or fee-only planner, doctors with lower levels of commitment can get a quick "lab report" from various on-line retirement planning engines such as those found at www.Fidelity.Com and www.Vanguard.Com. A middle ground, if you need more hand-holding, but not so much that you think you need a formal planner, is a semi-personalized "Retirement Planning Analysis" available for under $1000 from Vanguard.

Let's examine some of the other ways that you can re-balance or re-position your practice toward areas that are most profitable. Remember that at least in strict business terms, "winning" the ophthalmic profitability game shouldn't just be measured in total practice profits per year, but in the profit per surgeon hour. Seen in these terms, LASIK's allure has faded somewhat.

In the typical general practice, net surgeon profit per hour of professional time ranges from about $200 to $500. Before LASIK fees started to erode from a typical average price point of $1,600-$2,400 two years ago to about $1,100-$1,800 today (leaving out the steep discounters,) the profit per surgeon hour reached about $750—which is why everyone sprinted to LASIK training courses. Today, after accounting for steep marketing and technology costs and reduced professional fees, the typical profit per Lasik surgeon-hour has fallen to a number lower than that seen in efficient general/geriatric practices. The lesson? Don't become a LASIK surgeon because you think it will be a more profitable way to spend your day than as a general ophthalmologist. Actually, for the general ophthalmologist, the fastest way to higher profits is with a surgery center to vertically integrate your core cataract business.

Another useful metric of your service mix diversity and balancing is the so-called "average ticket," calculated by dividing monthly collections (for all medical and surgical care) by monthly total patient visits (both paid and unpaid operative care.) This and other statistics will be covered in much more detail in Chapter Nine, pages 125. But for the sake of the present discussion, consider the wide range of average ticket figures, and the impact of adding ancillary services:

- General ophthalmology practices without an optical, an ASC, or other forms of auxiliary revenue, typically have an average ticket of $150;
- For practices in especially challenging urban settings, where surgery yields are low due to an excess number of surgeons, the average ticket can range down to $125 or less. This is also the case for pediatric practices and for practices with a high proportion of low-cap-rate pre-paid patient care;
- Practices that add an optical component will typically see their average ticket (and collections) climb 15 percent to 25 percent. Average ticket figures then reach up to the $180 level in typical settings;
- Developing a surgery center, if executed and managed correctly, can easily add 50 percent to the revenue yield per average patient. The nuances of this are covered in Chapter Fourteen, pages 181;
- Adding one or more subspecialists to a general practice is a classic way to increase revenue yield per visit, and there can be an added boost of increased patient convenience and tenure.
- Retina and glaucoma are the common first additions. A general ophthalmology practice with any more than 50,000 patient visits a year can often support a full-time retinal surgeon; the thresholds can be much lower when a glaucoma specialist is added;
- Keep in mind that every setting is unique, and there can be special conditions in the market or in the practice that dampen the opportunity to diversify. Critically, the current physicians must be eager to delegate their subspecialty work; and
- To give you a sense of the revenue potential in these two areas, retinal surgeons typically have an average ticket of $200 to $450+ and glaucoma specialists enjoy an average ticket in the $180-$225 range.

Of course, revenue yield is just half of the picture. The net cash flow yields on these new lines of business can be excellent or poor depending on your execution, and what you end up paying for are new resources. Some optical shops generate 30 percent profit margins; some scrape along at 15 percent or less. Some surgery centers enjoy a 50+ percent profit margin. Multi-specialty centers with multiple users and poor cost containment limp along at 5 percent to 10 percent or less. Surgery centers that have been over-built to hospital/institutional standards are notoriously unprofitable.

What if you're a very average general ophthalmologist and don't have the threshold ambition or development capital to augment the practice's profit lines? There's still opportunity. Even if your case volumes fall below those needed to cash flow your own ASC, you can find a local facility to invest in and bring your cases. If you would rather not fuss with your own optical, you can contract with an independent optician or optometrist to establish a unit in your office, and arrange an appropriate lease payment or management fee. Your practice may not have enough glaucoma or retinal care to substantiate bringing on a full-time subspecialist—but you can still do much better economically than sending referrals to the local university department for free. You can simply bring in a part-time guest subspecialist who pays fair market rates for use of your facility and staff.

If you're a subspecialist reading this, you should see this opportunity from the flip side; there may be several colleagues in your service area who refer to you lightly now, who would have many more patients for you if you were in their office weekly or bi-weekly.

Unless you're nearing retirement, general economic cycles will influence your ophthalmic business affairs, both positively and negatively, several more times in the coming years of your career. Each successive cycle will force important decisions about re-balancing your service mix. Each of these decisions requires a rational fit between broad national market trends, your local conditions, your practice's economic demands, and as importantly, your professional standards and interests. Weaving these disparate threads into a viable practice fabric is at once the most challenging and the most satisfying part of owning an independent practice today.

Chapter Five: Questions That Can Improve Your Cash Flow and Your Bottom Line

Questions are like wonderful surgical instruments. In the hands of managers and practice owners, they can cut through the opaque outer layers of an organization and reveal the beating heart of operations. They reveal the vibrant elegance of a humming, well-run department, just as they reveal the decay and dysfunction of a department that is poorly run.

"Animal, mineral or vegetable?" The children's game of 20 questions comes in a grownup ophthalmologist's version that can boost your practice's strategic sharpness, operations and profits.

As a clinician, you long ago developed, refined, and memorized a question set to help you understand your patient's eye health. You don't ask every patient every question. But by the end of a typical clinic day, if we were to take an inventory, we'd see a score of questions that you've asked over and over again.

The clinical question set you use today is probably a lot shorter than the questions you used in the first year you practiced—you've learned what can be left out and what answers can allow a shortcut to the end of the exam. The most thoughtful doctors refine and personalize their clinical question sets to the very last day of their active practice.

You pose some of these questions to the patients directly or to their family members in the exam room. Some of the questions are posed to the ocular tissue you observe during a slit lamp examination or to the test results in your hands. Some of the questions are asked of an internal medicine colleague down the hall or a subspecialist consultant. Of course, some of the questions are muttered to yourself, when a real puzzler arises: "What in the world is going on here??"

The same game of "20 Questions" can be applied to the management side of your practice. Here's a starting point, with questions you can refine and apply daily, weekly, and in some cases monthly or annually in your practice. Some questions are micro, some macro. Some questions should be posed directly to management staff. Some should be posed to rank-and-file staffers. Some of the answers you get will speak for themselves and some should be cross-checked with outside experts.

20 Questions

1. Do we know what we want to do?

Too often, surgeons show up for work with goals that are no more defined than, "Let's make it through the day." It helps to deeply understand your personal goals and have these goals drive a formal strategic business plan. In the wise words of Henry David Thoreau, "Go confidently with your dreams. Live the life you have imagined." Ask yourself this question not just in the context of this week and this year, but in the context of your practice life. What big, hairy goals do you want to accomplish before you tear down the shingle you put up so proudly?

2. How cohesive is our practice team?

Does your practice have sufficient organizational "connective tissue" so that the lofty goals held by the doctor-owners are being translated completely into worka-day action? In the context of "cash flow," the language of these common goals should be numeric. It's often hard to get over the shyness and cultural taboos of discussing money, but in the highest-functioning practices, the managers know what the numbers are—cold—and what numbers they're trying to reach. Think about it. Why shouldn't the head tech know how many patients we aim to see in a typical month and how close we are to reaching our goals? If not only the head tech knows this, but the marketing manager, the front desk supervisor, and the billing manager, they'll have a whole new and improved basis on which to discuss the company's affairs.

3. Do we know what dimensions of our practice are growing, shrinking or staying the same?

Practice financial data is often too late, too scant, too short-term or not sufficiently segmented to back up your hunches. Bookkeeping controls must be in synch with the scale and financial challenges of your practice. The principals and the administrator of the practice, at the very least should know by rote the direction of all the major trendlines: revenue, expenses, patient volumes by doctor, new patient ratios, surgical density, waiting times for appointments and surgery, collection ratios, A/R ratios, etc.

4. Do we have control over the volume of patient visits and the mix and volume of surgical cases in our practice?

Rather than just taking what comes through the door, you should establish specific volume performance goals for the year, describing the number of new and total patients and mix of services you want to provide. You should then compare these figures monthly to actual performance, implementing whatever marketing actions are needed to meet your goals. The start of this process is believing you really can have an influence over what kinds of patients enter your practice—and you're not just waiting at the bottom of the chute for whatever drops into your lap.

5. Are there costs we could reduce without adversely impacting the quality of care we provide?

For example, replacing in-house patient transport vans with on-call taxis might still allow the desired end of serving indigent patients but at a lower cost and with greater flexibility to curtail services in the future if reimbursement trends erode further.

6. Do we need every person who is in the office today to serve today's patient loads?

Since much of any practice's costs are staff-related, look closely and often at your head counts. When you emerge from an exam room, are there routinely three technicians standing around? Most every time you walk into the insurance and billing office, are staff attending to the needs of the practice and patients, or huddled talking about their social lives? These are not questions posed to be vindictive, and some hang time is reasonable. But to survive in the world ahead of us, we're going to have to create practice cultures that value a strong work ethic and have no countenance for slackers.

7. Would slated cost containment efforts backfire and actually harm profitability?

For example, by reducing marketing costs $50,000 a year, you might reduce revenue by $100,000. By dismissing two techs, patient waiting time may climb to the point of reducing alumni referrals. Look ahead and try to forecast the potential unintended consequences of every cost-cutting effort.

8. Are there steps we could take to improve the quality of our patient care without adversely impacting profitability?

Remember that "quality" is not just clinical outcomes, but patient *perceptions*. For example, handing each patient an inexpensive printed fact sheet that describes his/her chief complaint and your treatment approaches would save some of the cost of having staff spend extra time educating each patient and would potentially improve patient compliance for better care. Everyone wins.

9. <u>When will we post charges for the services we provide to patients today?</u>
Too often, doctors concentrate on the over-90-day account column when the real problem is far earlier in the chain of events, for example, a bottleneck in the insurance department, generating a delay in claims submissions. Ask staff at the front lines about the time lag from service to posting. If the answer is anything more than 24 hours, ferret out the reasons. It may be that doctors hoard superbills and charts and don't complete their dictation or coding on time. It may be that the front desk staff can't multi-task as well as you might like and for a time—or forever—you would be better off batching charge posting in the insurance department.

10. <u>When will we submit claims for the services we provide our patients today?</u>
Ask staff what the time lag is from charge posting to claim submissions. If this is anything more than 24-48 hours, find out why. The most common reason given by the billing department is actually not, "We're running behind," but instead, "We've always just submitted claims weekly. What's the big deal? It doesn't hold things up that much."

11. <u>When will we get paid for the services we provide to patients today?</u>
How long does it take from the time we submit a claim to the time we receive payment? Is this in line with our colleagues in this area? If not, why? What happens—what are all of the nitty-gritty steps taken—when a check hits the door? Does it get deposited within a day or less, or does it languish five days until someone posts it?

12. <u>What percentage of the time do we get patients to pay the co-pays and deductibles and refraction fees for which they are responsible?</u>
The answer should be close to 100 percent. And yet, it's remarkable how many practices simply dismiss their patients without them paying a dime on the day of service. The same practices will then have staff spend months chasing those patients down. Not only does that practice delay cash flow, but the extra staffing costs to put out serial statements and place collections calls subtracts significantly from the money when it finally does arrive.

13. <u>How many hours do staff work every day, and how many hours are they paid to work?</u>
Practices, as they grow, can carry forward informal and sometimes even overly permissive wage and hour policies. This laxity can have a negative effect. Selected staff will abuse the system, claiming payment for extra time they didn't work each day. This costs the practice real dollars, and worse, leads to lower morale among the non-abusers. Overtime can get out of control. And valid claims can be made against the practice for violating labor laws.

14. Could we have seen more patients in the clinic today or performed more surgical cases?

Most surgeons end their work days with a cushion of unsold "inventory." It may not bother you that a few no-shows leave you time to read the paper. But remember that marginal, incremental revenue represents the bulk of your profits, since fixed costs are already covered. Just three missed exams a day in a typical solo practice can trim more than $50,000 from your annual income.

15. If we ended the day providing less care—doing less work—than was possible, what could we do to improve?

Giving yourself a five-figure annual raise could be as simple as adding one or two slots to the appointment template, or calling patients 24 to 48 hours ahead of their appointment to reduce no-show rates.

16. If we saw all the patients or performed all the cases we thought we were capable of, what's holding us back from doing *more*?

If growth is a goal, look for opportunities to increase everyone's productivity. Potential answers lie in back-office technology, increased tech training, or increased physician delegation of care to optometrists. Note that you may not want more patients packed into the day, but an extra hour to spend with your family. Knowing your goals is the start to achieving them.

17. Do we extract a full measure of value from every staff resource in the practice?

Look at the front desk. Are receptionists hanging out waiting for the next patient to arrive, or are they prepping the next day's charts? You wouldn't put your investment portfolio in an interest-free checking account—why would you let a $15-an-hour member of your staff not *continuously* earn their keep? Prepare a collateral/elective duties list for every department and let staff know you expect this list to be worked on during light days.

18. Do we extract full value from every *other* resource in the practice?

Satellite offices or surgical facilities left vacant most of the week were affordable in an era of $1,500 cataracts. Today, all offices should be open full-time, and an increasing number of practices have added evening and weekend hours to extract a full measure of value from fixed asset costs. Satellite offices can no longer be accumulated like vacation homes or sports cars. They must be put to good use.

19. Are we even in the right business? Do we have the right business model?

Have we gone too far to turn a cataract practice into a LASIK practice, now that fees for refractive surgery have fallen and volume growth has stagnated in some markets? Have we considered ourselves a surgical practice only and missed primary care and optical dispensing opportunities? Should we combine with compatible colleagues in town and form a larger group that can more efficiently spread fixed overhead?

20. What's our exit or succession plan?

Smaller practices have an easy answer: Sell to another practice in the community, or bring a successor surgeon in a few months before retirement. Large and "mega" practices have a more complex challenge. Since the demise of corporate management companies, and hospitals backpedaling from '90's merger mania, divestiture options have narrowed. For these large practices, succession planning should be nailed down at least five years before the retirement of the most dominant provider.

In Summary

In the heat of daily battle, few surgeons and few managers take the time to ask these questions, much less act on the answers. Your practice—in both clinical and business dimensions—is the most important "patient" to which you provide care. It's certainly the most demanding. Learn to ask the right questions every day and you will improve your organization's treatment plan and prognosis.

Section II: Torrents

Doing More and Getting Paid for What You Do

"All progress is based upon a universal desire on the part of every organism to live beyond its income."

Samuel Butler

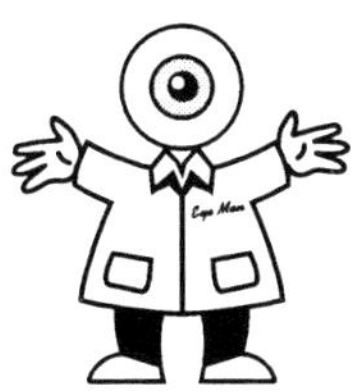

Chapter Six: Documentation and Billing Tips

Maintaining Adequate Cash Flow Involves More Than Just Your Accounts Receivable Department

The largest source of cash flowing through America's ophthalmology practices comes from just one place: Medicare. One of the basic premises you face when you deal with the government is to understand that payments received from Medicare are interim payments only. If Medicare audits you, they might ask you to repay some of that money should the service be deemed not medically necessary or incorrectly billed. Just because Medicare initially paid the service doesn't always mean the payment is correct.

In billing claims to Medicare, it is important to keep this in mind. You should always make sure your Medicare claims are submitted correctly and as error free as possible. Clean claims, as Medicare calls them, also help expedite payments and help keep a practice's revenues at an optimal level.

As a Medicare provider, like it or not, you are also bound by all kinds of government guidelines and regulations. Most of these guidelines pertain to documentation, coding, and billing Medicare claims. How you comply with these guidelines will determine whether or not you get to keep the interim payments you receive from Medicare. Properly documenting your patient medical records can help accomplish this goal.

Adequate Documentation Is Critical

With the Centers for Medicare and Medicaid Services (CMS) requesting that Medicare carriers increase their level of audit activity to recoup erroneously paid claims, there is a real need to re-visit the basics of chart documentation. This "getting back to the basics" will, in part, ensure that you will not suffer a Medicare audit (or at least will lessen the potentially financial devastation that may result from an audit).

Before we discuss the documentation requirements, however, there are some medical and legal factors that must also be considered when documenting a medical chart.

- **Quality of patient care**. If previous examinations do not contain the information that is required to make sound medical judgments, the patient may suffer as a result of unwarranted—and perhaps risky—tests being performed.

- **Medical and legal implications**. In the event of a malpractice complaint, what is, or is not, documented in the chart will be a crucial determinant of the final outcome.

- **Medical Necessity**. If the chart does not adequately support the medical necessity of the procedure or surgery to be performed, Medicare could find that the patient was put at undue risk due to the lack of medical necessity for the surgery. This could lead to suspension or revoking of one's medical license.

For non-Medicare patients, many third party payers require prior authorization before performing medical treatment or surgery and conduct utilization review of questionable physician practices. Adequate chart documentation is a key factor in determining if proper authorization is granted and if any action might be taken as a result of utilization review.

Is there any one "right" way to document a patient chart? Not really. You simply need to choose the medical charting format that will suit the unique individual needs of your particular practice. The S.O.A.P. charting technique that is taught in medical schools is the generally accepted documentation method preferred by Medicare auditors.

The four basic S.O.A.P. elements are:

S - Subjective (reason for visit);
O - Objective (services and tests performed);
A - Assessment (findings, diagnostic impressions, etc.); and
P - Plan (treatment and return check).

The ***Subjective*** section of the chart must always record the purpose of the patient's visit. The chart entry should include the patient's name and date of the visit; chief complaint, symptom, or reason for the visit; and the pertinent medical history as appropriate for each visit.

The ***Objective*** section is devoted to the services performed during the examination. This will support what you did during the visit; i.e., content of service. The ***Objective*** entries should include the findings obtained from the ocular examination, any tests ordered, and results of any special diagnostic tests performed. This portion of the chart is also where we apply the following adage:

IF IT ISN'T IN THE CHART
IT WASN'T DONE!

The ***Objective*** entry of the chart also provides the person that completes the superbill with the data necessary to select the proper procedure codes to be billed. In order to ensure that all documentation is complete, we recommend the use of preprinted examination sheets to include space for at least the following:

- unaided visual acuity
- cycloplegic visual acuity
- manifest refraction acuity
- glare test results
- intraocular pressure
- drops used for dilation and the time instilled
- confrontation/gross visual fields
- extra-ocular motility
- pupil evaluation
- external (lids, lashes and lacrima)
- slit lamp (conjunctiva, cornea, anterior chamber, angles, lens, vitreous)
- space for gonioscopy drawings
- routine ophthalmoscopy, c/d ratios
- space for extended ophthalmoscopy drawings
- mental status

The ***Assessment*** entries provide the recording of the decision you reached during the course of the examination. The ***Assessment*** should include indication of progress, a listing of each separate problem or diagnosis, conclusions, and resolution of findings. This is the final diagnosis you assign which represents the condition responsible for the patient's problems. This may or may not be directly related to the patient's expressed complaint. If no support can be found for the patient's complaint, you should note this as well. The findings will support the recommendations you make to the patient regarding proper follow-up care or surgical intervention.

As a reminder, when using evaluation and management codes, documentation of "rule out" conditions and treatment options considered but not recommended should be noted here.

The ***Plan*** section of the chart provides the treatment plan recommended to the patient to correct, alleviate, or further delineate the conditions recorded in the assessment. The ***Plan*** entry should include management options considered but not chosen, a list of recommendations, treatment planned, medications prescribed with dosage and regimen, consultations or referrals with reason recommended, patient education, reason for diagnostic services, and anticipated patient return for further treatment. The information you document in the ***Plan*** entry also provides an audit trail to support the medical necessity for any follow-up visits or reexamination of the patient.

When documenting any patient chart, the content of the chart should be very detailed and contain notations of the findings from each step performed during the examination. Abnormal findings as well as normal findings must be recorded. Remember, you cannot over-document.

Remember, too, that you should use clear language and avoid any vague references when you document patient charts. Write legibly, and use drawings or pictures where needed. We also recommend that you use only standardized abbreviations. We had a practice contact us recently about a huge refund request they had received from Medicare. In reviewing the charts, we noticed the doctor had used her own non-standard abbreviations. This is not a problem other than she neglected to send a copy of her abbreviations to Medicare along with the requested charts. As a result, the Medicare auditor could not read the chart and denied a lot of services that were legitimate. If you do use non-standard abbreviations, just be sure to provide Medicare (or any third party payer) with a legend of the specialized abbreviations when submitting requested medical records.

Medicare 101—Getting Back to the Basics

There are also some basic Medicare 101 principles you should know. For instance, Medicare only pays for services that are deemed to be medically necessary, medically justified, and medically reasonable—the 3M's of Medicare. Medicare will not pay for services that do not meet these criteria, are determined to be for the patient's personal comfort, are refractive in nature, or are services classified as "routine." Let's examine the 3M's a little more closely:

- **Medical Necessity** - Services that are consistent with the symptoms or diagnosis of the illness or injury under treatment and determined to be necessary and consistent with generally accepted professional medical standards (not experimental or investigational);

- **Medical Justification** - Services which are not furnished primarily for the convenience of the patient, the attending physician, or another physician or supplier; and
- **Medical Reasonableness** - Services that are furnished at the most appropriate level and can be provided safely and effectively to the patient.

In order to ensure that the services you perform are medically necessary, Medicare carriers perform both pre-payment and post-payment utilization review of claims submitted for payment. During an audit, if the medical necessity of the service is not substantiated by the medical records, the service is denied and a refund will be requested. The difference between a denial and a request for a refund is if the physician's records are thoroughly and appropriately documented.

Before moving on to the documentation criteria, there is one more important principle you need to remember:

> The Medicare Carriers Manual §2320 states that coverage of eye examinations performed by an ophthalmologist or optometrist is dependent on the purpose of the examination rather than on the ultimate diagnosis of the patient's condition. When a beneficiary has a complaint or symptom of an eye disease or injury, the services (except for eye refractions) are covered regardless of the fact that only eyeglasses were prescribed. However, when a beneficiary has no specific complaint, the examination is not covered even though the doctor discovered a pathologic condition.

Ophthalmology and optometry are the only two specialties that must comply with this guideline. This is because ophthalmologists and optometrists perform two types of eye examinations—medical and refractive. Medicare does not cover refractive exams, so the patient chart must document a patient complaint, symptom, or previously diagnosed condition in order for the service to be covered. To ensure that a service is not determined to be refractive in nature or a routine visit, it is your responsibility to obtain a chief complaint or note in the chart the medical reason for the visit.

How is this best accomplished? Usually the ophthalmic technician obtains this information from the patient or by reviewing the previous visit documented in the patient's chart even before the doctor enters the room. If the previous visit indicates a return check for "cataracts," then the subjective entry would indicate this as the reason for the visit. If the patient is a new patient or is there off-cycle, then every effort should be made to obtain a chief complaint from the patient. In this regard, the technician plays a very important role in the documentation process for an eye examination.

The documentation of the chief complaint for a new patient must note the specific problem that brought the patient to the office. The chief complaint is critical for a new patient encounter. Without it, Medicare will determine the services to be routine and not billable. Most offices prefer the use of a patient-completed preprinted history form to collect the necessary data from the patient. Or, the technical staff may query the patient prior to the history taking.

For an established patient, the reason for the visit can be a complaint, a symptom, or follow-up of a previously diagnosed medical condition. As previously stated, the technician should first look at the Plan entry of the previous visit to see if this is a scheduled visit (i.e., cataract check, IOP check, etc.). If it is, the technician would enter this information in the Subjective portion of the chart before asking the patient if he or she has any new problems the doctor needs to know about.

If the patient is a surgical candidate, the chart must also document a functional lifestyle impairment that was obtained from the patient to help support the medical necessity for any impending surgery. During the initial taking of the patient's medical history by the technician, a notation must be made of any comments the patient makes relating to changes in lifestyle or activities he or she no longer performs such as:

- Can't drive at night
- Can't read labels on medicine bottles
- Can't read
- Can't enjoy TV

This information is usually collected on a patient-completed questionnaire. Patients then assess their own lifestyle impairments by listing activities or hobbies they can no longer perform because of their failing eyesight.

Is a lifestyle impairment required for all surgical procedures? No, just cataract, YAG laser capsulotomy, and blepharoplasty. This additional documentation helps support the medical need for these surgeries as required by Medicare. Remember also:

- Functional impairment must be documented for **each** eye. Most practices believe that obtaining functional lifestyle impairment prior to the first eye surgery is sufficient. This is not true.

- Surgery on the second eye must be justified by the same criteria as for the first eye. In other words, functional impairment and vision requirements must be obtained again prior to the second eye surgery. And, there must be slit lamp entries to support the fact that the previously operated eye is "healed and stable."

Additional Documentation Guidelines

(1) Ophthalmic Exams
Most Medicare carriers require that comprehensive eye examinations, codes 92004 and 92014, be dilated and 8-9 elements documented. In addition, you must initiate a diagnostic or therapeutic treatment program. This can be as simple as a prescription for new glasses, a change in medications, or referral to another doctor. "Continue present meds" or requesting the patient to return merely for observation does not constitute the initiation of a diagnostic or therapeutic treatment program.

An intermediate eye examination, codes 92002 or 92012, usually contains 7 or fewer exam elements. We recommend no fewer than 3 elements. Without these elements, you would have to down code the service to an evaluation & management (E/M) service.

The required elements of an eye examination are:

- Visual acuity (not to include determination of refractive error);
- Measurement of intraocular pressures (except in children and patients with trauma or infectious disease);
- Gross visual field testing (confrontation visual fields);
- Examination of ocular adnexa including lids (e.g., ptosis or lagophthalmos), lacrimal glands, lacrimal drainage, orbits, and pre-auricular lymph nodes;
- Test ocular motility including primary gaze alignment;
- Inspection of bulbar and palpebral conjunctivae; and
- Examination of pupils and irises including shape, direct and consensual reaction (afferent pupil), size (e.g., anisocoria), and morphology.

Slit lamp examination of:

- Corneas including epithelium, stroma, endothelium, and tear film;
- Anterior chambers including depth, cells, and flare; and
- Lenses including clarity, anterior and posterior capsule, cortex, and nucleus.

Ophthalmoscopic examination through dilated pupils (unless contraindicated) of:

- Optic discs including size, C/D ratio, appearance (e.g., atrophy, cupping, tumor elevation), and nerve fiber layer; and
- Posterior segments including retina (vitreous, macula, periphery) and vessels (e.g., exudates and hemorrhages).

Be sure to check with your Medicare carrier for specific documentation and billing guidelines for intermediate and comprehensive eye examinations. Most Medicare carriers also expect to see at least one element of the slit lamp examination and one element of the fundus examination in order to distinguish it from the E/M services. Not meeting these specific criteria could result in a refund request in the event of an audit.

(2) Evaluation & Management Services Versus Ophthalmic Examinations
The five levels of E/M services (codes 99201–99275) and the two levels of ophthalmic services (codes 92002–92014) give ophthalmologists an array of levels for coding their services. A good rule of thumb is that most ophthalmic examinations are best billed with the ophthalmic codes, either intermediate or comprehensive. The E/M codes should be used for consultations or for examinations that are performed on patients whose medical conditions warrant the E/M level of service.

In general, the documentation requirements for E/M services are more specific and extensive than for the ophthalmic codes. It should be noted that the higher level E/M codes, i.e., levels 4 and 5, are potential audit flag codes. We caution that these E/M services must contain the chart documentation to support billing this level of E/M service. Briefly comparing E/M and ophthalmic services:

- History - The higher E/M levels 4 and 5 generally require either a detailed or comprehensive history whereas the intermediate and comprehensive ophthalmic services require only a patient complaint and a history or interval history;
- Examination - Most ophthalmic examinations meet the detailed and comprehensive examination requirements for the higher level E/M services. If the services performed in an ophthalmic examination fall below that of an intermediate ophthalmic examination, then a lower level E/M service should be billed; and

- Medical Decision Making - Ophthalmic examinations only have to have a diagnosis and plan for treatment whereas the E/M services utilize four, progressively more involved levels of medical decision making ranging from straightforward to low, moderate, and high complexity.

We recommend you follow the 1997 E/M guidelines published by CMS because they are more favorable to ophthalmology. We also suggest the use of a forced-entry or check-off type chart sheet as opposed to a blank progress sheet. Forced-entry forms eliminate the chance of the carrier being unable to determine exactly what services were performed or documented.

Another thing to remember is that the medical record is frequently the key document in a medical malpractice lawsuit or OIG investigation, so before making any alterations to your medical records, make sure you do so legally. Altered records can lead to allegations of fraud and cover up and put the credibility of the entire document and the witness in jeopardy. It has been found that in malpractice suits where documentation and record keeping were judged inadequate, damages were paid in two-thirds of the cases. However, when documentation and record keeping were judged adequate, damages were paid in only one-third of the cases.

Do not attempt to erase, overwrite, obliterate, or cover with correction fluid. In case of an error, simply draw a single line through the erroneous statement and then initial and date it. Make sure that the erroneous entry remains legible. It is an appropriate procedure to indicate why the correction was made.

Make certain that all records are written legibly. All records should be written in ink with a ballpoint pen using black or blue ink. Just remember that blue ink does not copy well and could be an issue when copying records for an audit. Never use pencil and avoid markers, which may bleed through the page and obliterate entries on the reverse side. If a patient has an adverse reaction to a medication, note it and the subsequent treatment. Add an adverse reaction sticker to the patient's chart so that the same medication is not given again.

Finally, for group practices, we recommend you sign each entry with your first and last names and professional designation, and always include the date.

(3) Consultations

Since consultations, CPT codes 99241–99245, are reimbursed at a much higher rate than regular office visits, you should make every effort to ensure that the documentation and billing guidelines are followed so that these higher services can be billed. Not billing for any correctly documented consultations will result in a loss of income to your practice. Consultations are billable from outside referrals or from patients referred by a member of your group practice.

A consultation is distinguished from a visit because it is provided by a physician whose opinion or advice regarding a specific problem is requested by another physician or other appropriate source (unless it's a patient-generated confirmatory consultation).

- A request for a consultation and the need for the consultation must be documented in the patient's medical record.

- In a group practice, this can be part of a plan written in the requesting physician's progress note, an order in the medical record, or a specific written request for the consultation.

- A request for a consultation from outside the practice may be documented by a specific written request or if the consultant's record shows a specific reference to the request.

After the consultation is provided, the consultant must prepare a written report of his or her findings, which is provided to the referring physician.

- In a group practice, the report may consist of an appropriate entry in the common medical record. We recommend that the requesting physician review and initial the entry, or a separate letter can be written.

- When the request for a consultation is from outside the practice, the consultant must prepare a separate document (letter) to communicate the findings to the requesting physician.

When can you tell if this is a referral for a consultation or simply a transfer of care? A transfer of care occurs when the referring physician transfers the responsibility of the patient's complete care (does not ever expect to see the patient again for that problem) to the receiving physician at the time of the referral. When a transfer of care occurs, the receiving physician would report a new or established patient visit, not a consultation.

A physician consultant may initiate diagnostic and/or therapeutic services at the initial consultation or a subsequent visit. Subsequent visits should be reported as an established patient office visit or subsequent hospital care, depending on the setting.

If an optometrist or general ophthalmologist from outside the practice identifies a cataract and refers the patient to the cataract surgeon, the surgeon can bill a consultation. In other words, if the patient's overall eye care is never completely transferred to the consultant, the receiving physician can bill a consultation as long as all the criteria for a consultation have been met. However, if an optometrist or general ophthalmologist in a group practice has identified a cataract, performed the majority of surgical work-up, and then merely sends the patient to the surgeon for the surgery, it is our opinion that a consultation should not be billed.

Remember also, in a group practice there is generally no medical necessity for the consultant to repeat the entire work-up if the referring doctor just performed a complete examination. The consultant is usually only reviewing the specific problem, and Medicare would deem it not medically necessary to bill a high level consultation for a referral within a group practice. Normally, code 99241 or 99242 is the level of intra-office consultation billed.

(4) Diagnostic Tests
Special diagnostic tests are covered only when the tests are ordered by the physician who is treating the patient. For example, A-scan, B-scan, endothelial cell counts, and so forth, performed as preoperative evaluations, must be ordered by the surgeon. If another member of your group practice other than the surgeon routinely orders all preoperative cataract testing, the insurance claim form must reflect the identity of the ordering/treating physician, not the performing or supervising physician. To support this billing method, clinics should develop a document that spells out the order for preoperative testing in which the treating physician is clearly identified. This will support the billing and provide a correct and appropriate audit trail.

The test must also be medically necessary before it can be billed to Medicare. The first place a carrier auditor might look for medical necessity of a diagnostic test is the chief complaint. If the patient has no complaints (i.e., there has been no noticeable change in the patient's vision since the last visit), auditors will look at the results of the general examination for the reason the test was ordered. How would you document medical necessity if the patient does not experience any obvious signs or symptoms as is the case with many posterior segment diseases? The examination should show that there are changes that require further study, and the appropriate diagnostic test can then be ordered. The changes from the last examination must be noted in the chart to support the need for the test ordered during the encounter. If there is an order for the test in the previous encounter, the reason must be clearly noted at that time.

In addition to a physician's order, most special diagnostic tests require a separate interpretation and report to support the medical necessity for the service billed. There is no national policy on what should be included in an interpretation and report. Based on our experience with Medicare carriers and chart audits performed by Medicare, we believe the following notations will provide Medicare with the needed information regarding an interpretation and report.

1) What was seen in the results of the test or what wasn't seen that was anticipated (e.g., glaucoma, macular degeneration),
2) What the finding suggests as to the status of the illness—improved or worsened (e.g., within normal limits, no change, worsened), and
3) What impact this may have on the treatment regimen of the patient (e.g., continue present meds, no treatment necessary, see Plan).

The interpretation and report can be documented in the chart with the use of a stamp with forced-entry fields, or you can include this information on a separate report.

Remember, too, that while the most commonly used diagnostic tests in ophthalmology do not require physician supervision, there are some tests that do require a physician to be present in the clinic or in the lane when the test is performed. For Medicare billing purposes an M.D., D.O., or O.D., meets the criteria of physician supervision. The different levels of supervision requirements are outlined below.

General Supervision - The procedure is furnished under the physician's overall direction and control, but the physician's presence is not required during the performance of the procedure. Under general supervision, the training of the non-physician personnel who actually performs the diagnostic procedure and the maintenance of the necessary equipment and supplies are the continuing responsibility of the physician.

76516 - A-scan
76519 - A-scan with IOL calculation
76529 - Foreign body localization
92060 - Sensorimotor exam
92065 - Orthoptic/pleoptic training
92081 - Visual field, limited
92082 - Visual field, intermediate
92083 - Visual field, extended
92135 - SLGT
92250 - Fundus photo
92270 - Electro-oculography
92275 - Electroretinography
92283 - Color vision
92284 - Dark adaptation
92285 - External photos
92286 - Specular microscopy (endothelial cell count)

Direct Supervision - In the office setting, means the physician must be present in the office suite and immediately available to furnish assistance and direction throughout the performance of the procedure. It does not mean that the physician must be present in the room when the procedure is performed.

76511 - A-scan echography
76512 - B-scan
76513 - Immersion B-scan
92136 - Ophthalmic biometry w/IOL power
92235 - Fluorescein angiography
92240 - Indocyanine-green angiography

Personal Supervision - A physician must be in attendance in the room during the performance of the procedure.

92265 - Needle oculoelectromyography

Be sure to check with your specific Medicare carrier for local medical review policies for documentation and coding guidelines for diagnostic tests. Remember also, for digital type tests where the results are kept on a diskette, you should annotate in the chart the specific disk and location where the results are stored. Most doctors will keep several days of film on one diskette. Without this notation, Medicare could allege that the test was not actually performed.

(5) Surgeries
Documenting office surgeries requires more than a notation in the chart that it was performed. At a minimum, you need a description of any type of anesthetic administered, the instrumentation used to perform the surgery, and a statement about the outcome. For example, when eyelash removal is performed, you should indicate "with forceps," for lesions, you need to mention the size before the excision. You should also indicate the eye (RT/LT), or E1-E4 for eyelid procedures.

Laser surgeries don't require as much documentation as major surgeries in the hospital or ambulatory surgery center (ASC). A simple forced-entry form or "stamp" in the patient's chart listing the procedure to be performed, the type of laser used and the settings, the number of shots or burns, any anesthetic used, and the eye involved will provide the needed documentation.

Major surgeries require a dictated operative report describing the actual preparation of the patient prior to the surgery, the intraoperative procedures performed by the surgeon, and any complications that occur during the procedure. We recommend that a copy of the operative report be kept in the patient's clinical chart. It acts as a quality control to let Medicare know the report was generated and prevents the carrier from making the determination that the service was not performed.

As stated earlier, the clinic chart for cataract, YAG laser capsulotomy, and blepharoplasty must contain a patient's functional lifestyle impairment to support the medical necessity for the surgery. Without this lifestyle impairment, Medicare will deny the claim and the ASC or hospital claim in a post-payment audit.

As you can see, documenting the patient chart plays an important role in your cash flow management. Without appropriate documentation to support the services you performed and billed to Medicare, you stand the risk of having to refund huge amounts of money to Medicare in the event of an adverse audit.

Patient Authorizations

Before a service is even rendered to a Medicare patient, there are certain patient authorization forms that must be signed. Even something as mundane as not obtaining the proper consent form can cause a refund request and an allegation of billing Medicare for services not authorized by the patient.

Beneficiary Lifetime Authorization

The basic Medicare requirement is that the beneficiaries sign all claims to indicate that they received the services and consent to the release of any medical records necessary to document the claims. There are two exceptions to this rule: If the patient is unable to sign the claim form, a relative, friend, or legal guardian may sign the form on the patient's behalf; and if you have the patient sign a "lifetime patient signature form" and keep it in the patient's permanent medical record. The lifetime authorization allows you to submit claims without obtaining individual patient signatures on each claim.

A patient signature form is mandatory for claims that are filed electronically but is required for paper claims as well.

- The one-time signature is valid for the lifetime of the patient. You are not required to update this form annually as some practices may think.

- "Signature on File" can then be entered in the signature field on the claim form. This negates the need to have the patient sign every claim.

- You must allow the patient to cancel the form at any time at his or her request. Some patients want their authorization canceled if they move or change doctors. You are required by Medicare law to comply with the patient's request.

- The form must be available for Medicare inspection upon request. As such, the form must be a permanent part of the patient's medical record.

Are patient signature forms really necessary? Doesn't Medicare just assume the patient has given me permission to file the claim since I performed the service? No, this is not true. In fact, if you can't provide a signed patient authorization upon request by Medicare, it can allege that the services you billed on that patient's behalf are fraudulent.

You must also obtain a patient authorization form for Medicare patients who have Medicare supplemental insurance benefits (Medigap). Since Medicare sends Medicare payment information directly to the Medigap insurers, an authorization form is required to release that information. The patient authorization form and the language required for Medigap crossover claims can be combined into one form.

Waiver of Liability Notices

In addition to the patient signature authorization requirement, there are three other forms called "advance notices" that must be presented to the patient before providing certain services:

Advance Beneficiary Notice (ABN). The most common waiver notice is the advance beneficiary notice for medical necessity waiver of liability. An ABN is needed for physician services, durable medical equipment (DME) supplies, and ASC services. When Medicare denies a service as "not medically necessary or reasonable," you cannot bill the patient for the service unless you had an ABN signed by the patient before the service was rendered.

See Figure 1 on the next page for services that might require an ABN due to limited diagnoses or special circumstances.

Figure 1

Procedures that could be denied as not reasonable and necessary:

CPT Code	Short Description
92020	Gonioscopy
92081–92083	Visual Fields
92135	Scanning Laser Glaucoma Test
92225–92226	Extended Ophthalmoscopy
92235	Fluorescein Angiography
92240	ICG Angiography
92250	Fundus Photo
92285	External Photography
15820–15823	Blepharoplasty
66984	Cataract with IOL implant
67901–67924	Ptosis Repair
76512	B-scan

- As of October 1, 2002, Medicare requires you to use Form #CMS-R-131, which can be downloaded from www.cms.hhs.gov. You can add the name and address of the practice, but the language of the form cannot be modified in any way, and a copy must be given to the patient immediately upon signing the form. The use of any other ABN could be considered invalid by Medicare.

The waiver of liability notice must be specific to that particular service, on that specific date, and should be a part of the patient's medical record. The reason shown on the statement must be concise and address the reason the claim might be denied (see Figure 2 below).

Figure 2

Waiver of Liability Statements

- Medicare usually does not pay for this many visits or treatments for this condition [*list the condition*].
- Medicare does not pay for this service [*list the service*] because it is a treatment that has yet to be proven effective (a special waiver for any experimental procedure also recommended).
- Medicare usually does not pay for this many services [*list the services with the frequency*] within this period of time.
- Medicare usually does not pay for more than one visit a day.
- Medicare usually does not pay for like services by more than one doctor of the same sub-specialty.
- Medicare may consider this procedure [*list the procedure*] to be cosmetic only and not medically necessary.
- Medicare does not pay for this procedure [*list the procedure*] for this condition [*list the condition*].

A general statement that does not identify the specific service and the specific reason is not a valid waiver as Medicare refuses to recognize the use of "canned" ABNs. You should never use a statement such as, "I never know whether Medicare will deny this payment," and never have the patient sign a blank or vague notice in anticipation of *possibly* performing a non-covered service at some undetermined future date.

The ABN is needed only if you intend to bill the patient for any denied services. When using an ABN, you must append the GA modifier to the CPT procedure code. This tells Medicare that a signed waiver is on file and the charge is expected to be denied. Failure to use the GA modifier will result in inappropriate beneficiary liability information printed on the patient's Explanation of Medicare Benefits (EOMB). In other words, the patient will be advised that he or she will not be liable for payment of the denied service.

The medical necessity waiver notice does not apply to any service that is always noncovered, such as refractions, spectacles for non-aphakic patients, or topical medications (see Figure 3 below).

Figure 3

Other Noncovered Items That Do Not Require Advance Notice

- Cataract sunglasses obtained in addition to the regular (untinted) lenses
- Scratch-resistant coating
- Contact lens cleaning solution
- Normal saline for contact lenses
- Low-vision aids used to maximize residual vision

There are no mandatory instructions from Medicare regarding advance notice for services that are specifically excluded from coverage. However, if the patient wants you to bill Medicare for a secondary insurance denial, there are two modifiers that must be used.

- GY modifier – Item or service statutorily excluded or does not meet the definition of any Medicare benefit. This modifier would be used for cosmetic or refractive surgery, for instance.

- GZ modifier – Item or service expected to be denied as not reasonable and necessary. This modifier lets Medicare know that you have no signed ABN on file and that you do not expect to bill the patient in the event the service is denied.

We believe it is prudent to make it standard protocol to provide each patient with a written notice when a non-covered service is to be provided. This will help to prevent unnecessary and unpleasant interaction with the patient when the bill comes. We also suggest you post a large-print sign in the waiting area stating that refractions are not covered by Medicare and are the patient's responsibility.

Financial Hardship Notice. Routinely waiving co-insurance and deductibles is prohibited under Medicare. When a participating agreement is signed with Medicare, you have indicated that you will accept Medicare's payment as payment in full for services you render to Medicare patients. In this regard, you must also make an attempt to collect any co-insurance and deductibles associated with these covered services.

Some patients, however, do not have secondary insurance coverage and just simply cannot afford to pay even the co-insurance and deductible amounts. In these instances, you can determine if the patient is considered a financial hardship case, and on occasion, agree to accept only what Medicare will pay in full. In the event this is true, you must have the patient sign a financial hardship waiver that attests he or she cannot afford any out-of-pocket expenses. The waiver must be kept in the patient's medical chart as proof of indigence.

Occasional waiver of co-insurance and deductibles such as this are not considered fraudulent. However, to make sure you don't run afoul of the Medicare rules governing routine waiver of co-insurance and deductibles, here are some guidelines you should follow:

- If your percentage of waivers is high (over 20 percent), appropriate action must be taken to limit the number of economic hardships granted.

- The criteria you use to judge a Medicare patient's ability to pay the deductible and co-payment must be objective and fair to all patients. The guidelines must also be applied consistently.

- There must also be a good-faith attempt to ascertain the patient's financial condition. The questions should be limited to determining the amounts and sources of the patient's income (e.g., Social Security, pension).

- A supervisory staff member should conduct the patient interview in a confidential manner. It should be made clear to the patient that the economic hardship is granted on an individual, as-needed basis only and that Medicare requires a determination of the patient's ability to pay.

- If a patient is to have surgery, you must make him or her aware of the hospital or ASC charges and that your economic hardship waiver does not include the hospital or non-physician owned ASC charges.
- Review the financial hardship waiver periodically with the patient, especially if unusual or extenuating circumstances exist, to determine if the economic hardship still applies.

Some state medical associations have specific criteria for determining a patient's financial status and ability to pay. You should contact your state society and ask if they have guidelines available and make sure your financial hardship waiver is in compliance with state laws.

Deluxe Frames Waiver. There is another waiver you will need to obtain from your patients if you own an optical shop—the Deluxe Frames Waiver. Under Medicare rules, only standard eyeglass frames (costing about $50) are considered for reimbursement. Should the patient choose more expensive deluxe frames (costing more than $50), the cost difference for the deluxe frames is not covered by Medicare.

In order to collect the difference in cost between the standard frames and the deluxe frames from the patient, you would need to have the patient sign a Deluxe Frames Waiver so there is no misunderstanding about the portion of the frames that Medicare will cover. Without the signed waiver, you cannot collect the differential from the patient.

Since deluxe frames are excluded from Medicare coverage and not denied based on medical necessity, it is our opinion that you would continue to use the Deluxe Frame Waiver as stated above and not the new ABN form for this purpose. However, if your Medicare carrier should instruct you to do otherwise, you should follow its directions.

The above advance notices should always be given to your patients when you have some genuine doubt regarding the likelihood of Medicare payment. If you do not intend to collect for the service from the patient, then advance notices are not necessary. A sample patient authorization and sample advance notices can be found in the Appendix Three of this book.

Additional Coding Tips

(1) Refractions
Refractions are not included in any level of office visit and are excluded from Medicare payment. Typically, refractions are performed for the purpose of prescribing lenses and include specification of lens type (monofocal, bifocal, other), lens power, axis, prism, absorptive factor, impact resistance, and other factors; when documented as such, the refraction, code 92015, is billable to the patient.

If a prescription for lenses is not the intent and the refraction is used to determine the patient's best corrected visual acuity as an element of the examination, then most physicians choose not to bill the patient for the refraction. They consider this an integral part of the pre-operative or post-operative examination and not billable separately because a refraction (for the purpose of prescribing lenses) is not performed.

The above is merely our suggestion on the subject of when to bill or not bill for refractions. Ultimately, it is the physician's decision when to bill the patient for this Medicare-excluded service. You should also keep in mind that collecting refractions at the time of service helps improve cash flow.

(2) Physician's Signature
Should the physician sign each and every chart? The only reference Medicare has made regarding physician signature is found in the documentation requirements for billing evaluation & management (E/M) services which indicates that the physician performing the service must be identified. This is particularly important in group practices where the patients are seen by more than one doctor. Some

Medicare carriers, however, have published newsletter articles indicating their desire to have the physician sign each and every chart. Another consideration in having the physician sign the chart is for risk management purposes. A majority of medical malpractice insurance carriers require that each chart entry be signed or initialed by the physician.

(3) Superbills

Do you use one main superbill for all your services? Or do you separate retina, glaucoma, cataract, services? Most group practices find it easier to use separate superbills per specialty. Regardless of the type of superbill you use, make sure the diagnosis and CPT codes are updated annually. List only the most common procedures performed with blanks in each section for writing in other procedures. Some practices also believe it is better to have exams and diagnostic tests on one superbill and surgery on another. The design of your superbill is your choice; you just need to make sure it adequately includes all the services and diagnosis codes that are common to your practice.

Medicare does not require physicians to sign the superbill. Check your state medical and other insurance requirements before making this decision.

(4) Maintaining Adequate Practice Fees

One of the most frequently asked questions we receive is whether or not a practice can maintain separate fee schedules—one for Medicare and another for commercial insurance. Two separate fee schedules are permitted under Medicare provided the commercial insurance fee schedule is not less than Medicare's allowable for any one service. You may also keep separate fee schedules for optometrists in your practice as long as their charges are not less than Medicare's allowed amount.

Charging commercial or private pay patients less than you charge Medicare patients could result in a Medicare determination that you are discounting these patients and not Medicare. Medicare makes an exception for contracted groups of people such as HMOs and PPOs. If you agree to a set payment under one of these policies, you are not violating Medicare's assignment agreement.

You should revise your fees on an annual basis to avoid any underpayments from Medicare. The Medicare Fee Schedule is usually updated in November of each year and forwarded to you in a newsletter. Most practices keep their fees at about 30–50 percent above Medicare's allowable to also cover any higher commercial insurance payments. Some practices charge about 120 percent above Medicare's allowable.

Remember, as a Medicare participating provider, you can charge whatever you want as long as it equals or exceeds Medicare's allowable. Charging less than Medicare's allowable will result in an underpayment since Medicare pays the lower of the two—your charge or their allowable. Non-participating providers may only bill Medicare patients 115 percent above Medicare's allowable for that service.

(5) Correct Coding Initiative
One of the most critical changes to occur in Medicare billing in a long time was the implementation of the Correct Coding Initiative (CCI) in 1996. CCI was developed to accurately report and uniformly pay for physicians' services under the Medicare physician's fee schedule. Many practices still do not understand the edits or the reasons behind them.

By definition, the CCI edits bundle together those separate, though integral, services of a procedure into one comprehensive service. The comprehensive procedure is one that best describes the total service performed during that session. The CCI edits apply to the same physician, performing all services on the same patient, on the same day.

A complete list of CCI edits can be viewed and downloaded from the CMS website at www.cms.hhs.gov. It is critical that these edits be made available to the coding staff because without the current edits, they cannot effectively do their job.

Claim Form Submission

Now that you know the basic documentation requirements and the rules regarding advance notices, you are ready to file your claims to Medicare. If you currently file paper claims, you should consider very seriously switching to electronic claims because it can enhance your cash flow management and make life a whole lot easier for you and your staff. The benefits of electronic billing include the following:

- Your Medicare Part B claims process faster and you are reimbursed sooner, improving your cash flow. Payment for electronic claims may be released after 13 days; payment for paper claims must be held for 27 days;

- Your mailing and administrative costs are significantly reduced, thus improving cash flow;

- Fewer claims are returned with development letters, saving your staff time and effort;

- You have better control over filed claims. The data you enter into your system goes directly into the Medicare claims processing system exactly the way you send it; there is no need for intermediate data entry. A response report lets you know that Medicare's computer system has received your data;

- The patient account number appears on every Remittance Notice you receive, which reduces time spent locating payment posting information;

- Most Medicare carriers provide on-line inquiry, which allows easy access to claims status. If available, this information is obtained through dial-up capabilities using software that is provided at no cost and is compatible with your computer; and

- Most Medicare carriers provide ongoing customer support through an electronic claims processing help line.

Although electronic billing is the recommended optimum method for filing Medicare claims, if you are not equipped to file claims electronically, there are other options available to you.

You may have heard about optical character recognition (OCR). OCR is a technology some Medicare carriers use which permits the scanning and capture of printed data to be input directly into Medicare's computers. Medicare carriers use OCR to scan and lift information printed on the CMS-1500 claim form. OCR claims are subject to the 27-day payment floor. Only electronically filed claims have a reduced payment floor of 13 days.

Through the use of OCR, claims are entered into the processing system more rapidly than paper claims are entered. In addition to the speed of entry and reduction of handling time, the use of OCR reduces administrative costs and minimizes the manual intervention required to correctly process your Medicare Part B claims. Only the current CMS-1500 claim form with red dropout ink is acceptable for OCR. However, OCR is not the preferred way of submitting claims, and not all carriers have the capability.

Electronic funds transfer is another option Medicare uses for payment of claims. Matching EOMBs to actual payments can be a nightmare for a lot of computer systems, however. Be sure your computer system does not sabotage the benefits of electronic deposits before you agree to this method of payment.

CMS-1500 Claim Form Instructions

Whether you file claims on paper or via electronic submission, knowing how to file a CMS-1500 claim form properly is essential. Submitting properly completed claims to Medicare will allow faster reimbursement and avoid denials in a post-payment audit (see Appendix Three). The following tips should help ensure the claims you file to Medicare are accurate and timely.

- The patient's name and HIC# must be entered correctly. This must be entered exactly as shown on the patient's Medicare card. Any other name or HIC# will cause unnecessary denials or erroneous payments.
- Provider number, UPIN, and the Tax ID number must be correct. Errors in these fields could result in the wrong provider being paid.
- Items 3, 9b, and 11a must have 8-digit dates (MM/DD/CCYY).
- Item 17 and 17a must include the name and UPIN of the referring doctor for consultations and diagnostic tests. Without this information on the claim form, the claim is returned unprocessed.
- Item 24a, Date(s) of Service, should be the date the service is performed, not the date the service is posted in the financial record. In an audit, a Medicare carrier's request for medical records might not coincide with the appropriate date. Enter either a 6-digit (MM/DD/YY) or 8-digit (MMM/DD/CCYY) date for each procedure, service, or supply When "from" and "to" dates are shown for a series of identical services, enter the number of days or units in Column 24g.
- Item 24b, Place of Service, must be "11" for office, "24" for ASC, "31" for skilled nursing facility, and "12" for DMERC claims. Misuse of these codes can affect the amount of payment.
- Item 24c, Type of Service, is no longer required for Medicare claims. However, if your computer system still includes this information, it is not going to cause a denial.
- Item 24d, Procedures, Services, or Supplies, must include the appropriate CPT or HCPCS code. Enter the specific procedure code without a narrative description. However, when you enter an "unlisted procedure code" or a "not otherwise classified" (NOC) code, include a narrative description in Item 19 or EMC equivalent. Otherwise, an attachment must be submitted with the claim.
- Item 24e, Diagnosis Code, shown on the claim form must be documented in the chart. If it isn't, you have filed a fraudulent claim. Enter only one reference number per line. When multiple services are performed, enter the primary reference number for each service, either a 1, 2, 3, or 4. The diagnosis must be in the form

of ICD-9-CM codes at their highest level of specificity. You must use the 4- and 5-digit codes, when available, that most exactly categorize the patient's illness or condition. There are some 3-digit diagnosis codes that apply to ophthalmology, but not many. Code the reason for the visit in box 21 of the CMS-1500 using an appropriate ICD-9 code. The patient's complaint or final diagnosis should be included on the second line of box 21.

- Item 24g, Days or Units, is most commonly used for multiple visits, units of supplies, or anesthesia minutes. If only one service is performed, the numeral 1 must be entered. For anesthesia, show the elapsed time (minutes) in Item 24g. Convert hours into minutes, and enter the total minutes required for this procedure.
- Item 24k, Reserved for Local Use, must show the individual PIN of the provider performing the service in a group practice. Otherwise, leave blank. In the case of a service provided incident to the service of a physician or non-physician practitioner, when the person who ordered the service is not supervising, enter the PIN of the supervisor in Item 24k.
- Item 32 must contain the name and address of the location where the service is rendered. This substantiates the place of service and confirms when a HPSA bonus can be made.

If services are furnished on and after October 1, you have until December 31, two years later, to file a claim to Medicare. However, by law, if you do not file claims within 12 months of the date of service, you will be assessed a 10 percent reduction in payment. If no claim at all is filed for the beneficiary when the services are possibly covered under Medicare, sanctions can be imposed.

For the majority of ophthalmic practices, a vast percentage of the practice's revenue comes from Medicare. In order to capture your commercial payments in a timely manner as well, you need to verify other payer guidelines to avoid lost revenue.

Now that you know your responsibility when it comes to filing claims with Medicare, what is Medicare's responsibility in processing and settling a claim? The carrier has certain timeliness criteria for issuing notices and informing providers of its initial determination for the charges filed. The law, established in 1986, requires all carriers to process at least 95 percent of all "clean" claims received within 30 days.

The carrier must meet this "functional standard" during the CMS review of the carrier's performance. If the carrier does not process the claim and send a notice of a final determination to pay or deny within 30 days, it is required to pay interest if payment is due. The carrier cannot issue a payment before 13 days after receipt of the claim if it is sent as an electronic media claim (EMC) or 27 days if filed by paper. Only clean claims are eligible for the interest payment.

Appeal Options

An appeal is a written or verbal request to Medicare to reconsider a claim due to dissatisfaction with the amount of payment or denial of payment of a Medicare claim. An individual who has a right to appeal is referred to as a "party."

Medicare providers need to be aware of the new appeals process effective January 1, 2006. The Medicare claims appeals process requires a new, second level in the administrative appeals process, called a "reconsideration," and is processed by Qualified Independent Contractors (QICs) instead of Medicare Fair Hearing Officers. The appeals process will now consist of five levels. Each level of appeal must be completed for each claim at issue prior to proceeding to the next level of appeal. No appeal can be accepted until an initial determination has been made for the claim. The five levels of appeal are (1) Redetermination, (2) Reconsideration, (3) Administrative Law Judge (ALJ) Hearing, (4) Departmental Appeals Board (DAB) Review, and (5) Federal Court (Judicial) Review.

The following is a brief overview of the more significant changes in the appeals process:

- All requests for the first level of appeal (redetermination) will need to be made in writing. Medicare will no longer be able to accept or process redeterminations over the telephone.

- All initial claims determinations, including those for overpayments and medical review, will need to go through the first level of appeal (redetermination), regardless of the amount in controversy. They will no longer go to the second level of appeal (hearing/reconsideration).

- A minor error or omission made in the billing of a claim may now be submitted for a clerical error reopening instead of having to be submitted as a redetermination. Requests for clerical error reopenings to correct the error or omission can be made in writing or over the telephone.

- The second level of appeal after the redetermination is also changing. It will no longer be processed as a hearing, but will now be referred to as a reconsideration. The $100.00 amount in controversy requirement is being eliminated. The second level of appeal that used to be conducted by carrier hearing officers will now be conducted by Qualified Independent Contractors (QICs).

Physicians and providers who wish to appeal an initial determination of a Medicare claim made by a Medicare carrier are encouraged to review the revised appeal guidelines. You can find this information on the CMS website. Failure to exercise the appeal rights under Medicare can adversely affect a practice's bottom line. It is very important for the billing office to pay attention to claim denials when posting the carrier determinations.

Appeal Process

The following outlines the steps in the Medicare appeal process:

- **Redetermination**
  - Performed by Medicare contractor
  - Time limit of 120 days from date of receipt of the notice of initial determination (Medicare Summary Notice [MSN] or Remittance Advice [RA])
  - Monetary threshold to be met or amount in controversy—none

- **Reconsideration**
  - Performed by the QIC
  - Case file prepared by the Medicare contractor and forwarded to the QIC
  - Medicare contractor may have effectuation responsibilities for decisions made by the QIC
  - Time limit of 180 days from date of receipt of the redetermination
  - Monetary threshold to be met or amount in controversy—none

- **Administrative Law Judge (ALJ)**
  - Case file prepared by the QIC and forwarded to the HHS Office of Medicare Hearings and Appeals (OMHA)
  - Medicare contractor may have effectuation responsibilities for decisions made at the ALJ level
  - Time limit of 60 days from the date of receipt of the reconsideration notice
  - Monetary threshold to be met or amount in controversy; at least $100 remains in controversy

- **Departmental Appeals Board (DAB) Review**
  - Contractor may have effectuation responsibilities for decisions made at the DAB level
  - Time limit of 60 days from the date of receipt of the ALJ hearing decision/dismissal
  - Monetary threshold to be met or amount in controversy—none

- **Federal Court (Judicial) Review**
  - Medicare contractor may have effectuation responsibilities for decisions made at the Federal Court level.
  - Time limit of 60 days from date of receipt of DAB decision or declination of review by DAB.
  - Monetary threshold to be met or amount in controversy; at least $1,050 remains in controversy.

The revisions to the appeals process do not change the available basis for claim denials. Medicare carriers may continue to deny claims on the basis that the item or service is not a Medicare benefit, or more precisely, that the item or service in question does not adhere to all the requirements set forth in the definition of the Medicare benefit. Rather, these revisions change the appeals status of providers and participating suppliers, allowing them to appeal all denials on their own accord.

Conducting Internal Audits

One of the most effective tools that can be utilized by a practice is to audit its own records. You should perform a routine chart audit as part of your on-going compliance program. (Please see Chapter Three on compliance programs.) It is also a good idea to have an outside firm audit the practice on a regular basis (every one or two years). The following guidelines should assist you in developing a good internal audit protocol that can then be supplemented with annual follow-up audits from an outside firm.

Set an audit schedule so that timing of charts is always different. For example, if there are five teams of auditors, each team should audit a different day of the week and a different area; e.g., diagnostic tests, anesthesia, level of service, etc. Then rotate the auditors so that each team becomes familiar with all aspects of the practice.

- Assignments for audit can be made on a monthly, weekly, or other basis. This is a great training tool for staff as well as a great promoter of better, more open communication between the front and back office personnel.

- No less than one full day's patient charts should be audited at each time. The documents needed for the audit are:

  - Patient chart;
  - Patient financial statement;
  - Explanation of Medicare Benefits (EOMB)/Medicare Summary Notices (MSN); and

    - Informed consent forms, operative reports, etc., as called for in the charts.

- Be very critical and carefully compare the codes billed to the actual CPT descriptions. Remember also, compliance is not just a Medicare issue anymore. With the fraud and abuse rules expanding into private insurance and managed care arenas, you should audit those records as well. Applying the basic Medicare rules to all lines of business should keep you in compliance.

- Physicians should participate in the audit process. *To establish a workable and effective internal audit team, there must be a commitment by everyone in the clinic.* Depending on the size of the clinic staff, teams should be assigned combining front office and back office staff to each team. This encompasses the total realm of medical and Medicare expertise in the practice.

- The sample audit form found in the Appendix can be used to assist you in the internal audit process on an ongoing basis. Following guidelines as simple as these can help avoid an adverse audit by Medicare and a possible refund request. Internal auditing and periodic on-site audits conducted by an outside firm are two more steps in the right direction for optimizing and maintaining adequate cash flow for your practice.

When the internal audit is completed, a brief summary report needs to be prepared and presented during full staff meetings. Trends need to be developed to get an overall measurement of the effectiveness of the audit for eliminating problem areas. Suggestions for corrective actions should be solicited from physicians and staff so that you can be sure they understand how the audit process is working. For instance:

- Do superbill problems cause a chain reaction of bad billing all the way through the practice?
- Are there claim delays because one doctor doesn't dictate operative reports on time?
- Does the technical staff document each diagnostic service performed?
- Are chief complaints properly obtained and entered into the charts?
- Are functional impairments obtained prior to cataract, YAG laser capsulotomy, or blepharoplasty surgery?

After the priorities are made, begin implementation of corrective actions. Assign certain personnel to check superbills and EOMBs/MSNs at the end of each day. Work with those physicians who do not spend enough time in their offices dictating. Be sure they have the time away from appointments to get this task accomplished. Assign a front office person to report to you on his or her findings from the EOMB/MSN monitoring process.

Then, TRACK, TRACK, TRACK!! A common problem in implementation of corrective actions is failure to track the results. To be successful, all persons responsible for specific tasks must be held accountable for their part. Conduct personal interviews in order to monitor each person's progress.

Hold staff meetings and communicate the results of internal monitoring and tracking in order to develop consistency among staff members and get feedback from those who are part of the team. Remember, your ability to work more efficiently, to build an efficient staff, and to stay on top of changes will determine the compliance success of your practice.

Mandatory Office Tools

Every insurance clerk in the practice, as well as the compliance officer, should be familiar with Medicare payment rules, the *Medicare Carriers Manual* (Part 3), and carrier coverage and payment policies. Most carriers have web pages on the Internet that contain current medical policies that should be reviewed for updates. Almost any large public library will have access to the government publications such as the *Medicare Carriers Manual*. Another way to get information on coverage, documentation, and payment criteria is to attend carrier-sponsored seminars and professional society seminars on changes in Medicare guidelines.

The insurance/billing department should *never* use outdated CPT or diagnosis code manuals. When new manuals are published, usually in the fall, make every effort to obtain at least one copy for the office before the New Year. The manual can be checked against the fee slips for necessary changes in codes for the procedures or diagnoses. Often, small changes are made in definitions that affect how a service is billed.

Other documents that must be regularly reviewed are the Correct Coding Initiative (CCI) edits, which are usually updated on a quarterly basis. These edits can be viewed and downloaded at www.cms.hhs.gov/physicians/cciedits/. Failure to be aware of the changes will result in lost revenue to the practice. A quick checklist of mandatory office tools can be found in the Appendix One.

Troubleshooting

In today's environment of reduced Medicare payments, practices can hardly afford the luxury of delayed payments or loss of revenues to which they are entitled.

Most Medicare carriers provide periodic updates in their newsletters about common claim errors that can be used by the practice to track these same problems.

Regardless of the type of information an office receives from Medicare or other primary sources of revenue, tracking and reporting systems should be developed and utilized on a monthly basis to determine the effectiveness of their own claim filing techniques. A lot of large clinics have quick and easy monitoring systems. If on Monday morning, the bank account is not at a certain level, they know there has been a glitch in the Medicare payment income. Audit trails are then followed to determine the nature of the problem. This can be effective only if the clinic is certain that there are no significant problems in its own claims filing process.

Effort should be made to ensure that claims are not filed with the following types of problems. These problems represent the top five billing errors for claim denials or delays in payment.

1) Billing for visits in the global fee period without modifier 24 and/or without documentation to support the use of modifier 24; i.e., proof that the condition necessitating the visit was not related.

2) Billing with invalid diagnosis codes or with a diagnosis code not covered for the procedure performed.

3) Payment previously made to another provider. This is a difficult situation to avoid since the prior visit may be unknown at the time of service. Proper patient inquiry at the time of the visit can help to eliminate this type of error.

4) Billing for surgery during a global fee period without a modifier. Modifier 58, 78, or 79 must be appended to surgical services performed during the global fee period, by the same surgeon, no matter how obvious it is that this surgical episode is not related to the global fee period.

5) Service billed is bundled into another service. This is a particularly troublesome issue since billing for a bundled service is prohibited.

Electronic claim submitters will receive quarterly or semi-annual reports from Medicare providing claim submission errors. Are these pieces of information important? YES!

Computer screens can and should be developed to keep these errors from occurring. Also, any denials for these reasons should be carefully researched to ensure the carrier did not make an error. They do make processing errors, and they are usually significant. If an error is detected, a telephone review should be initiated for correction to get the cash flow back on track. Once this is done, internal systems need to be developed to correct the problem. In many cases, these problems need to be corrected at the clinic even though the problem exists with the carrier. While this doesn't seem fair, it is most expedient to make the correction for the sake of future of cash flow.

Maintaining compliance and an adequate cash flow requires a concerted effort on the part of every physician and staff member. Implementing a strong reimbursement management approach with key objectives and goals just puts you one step ahead of the game. Flow charts outlining this approach can be found in Appendix Two.

Remember, the way to obtain the best cash flow is having checks and balances in place to ensure that you get to keep those interim payments in the event of a Medicare audit.

Chapter Seven:

Organizing Reception and Patient Accounts Management in Your Office for Improved Cash Flow

Superior Patient Accounts Work
Starts With Having The Right Staff

"Money is better than poverty, if only for financial reasons."
Woody Allen

Before digging into practical realities, let's engage in a little fantasy. Just imagine it was a perfect world, and patients routinely and cheerfully paid for their own eye care the same way they go through the checkout line at the grocery store. Or imagine eye surgeons were paid by the hour, with different billing rates based on experience, like lawyers and accountants. Imagine that the ophthalmic world was fully wired, and patients would simply swipe smart cards at various service stations in your practice, receive services, and send a bill to Medicare at the speed of light, as readily as happens when you buy a tank of gas.

And just imagine third-party payers reviewed claims and were actually helpful in pointing out mistakes and educating staff so you were paid fairly and promptly for your work. If any of these were the case, the typical clinic, with three or four doctors and a few million dollars in annual collections could get by with a single low-level billing clerk instead of two, three, or more resident experts.

Extrapolating any of these fantasies to the entire country, we might free up at least 10,000 workers in America in ophthalmology alone to directly help doctors and serve patients rather than having to spend their working lives so frustratingly, chasing down lost and missing payments.

Alas, we live with reality and not fantasy. As a result, we need to hire, train and supervise more than 10,000 people in ophthalmology so the doctors and everyone else on the team can get paid for their work.

Let's start with a few basics. In the typical setting, your patient accounts department needs one full-time staff member (one full-time equivalent or "FTE") for every $800,000 to $1.2 million in annual collections. This calculation includes everyone involved with posting charges, submitting claims, posting payments, resubmitting claims that had errors, submitting secondary claims, and following up with payers and patients when claims go unpaid.

Practices with a very high average revenue yield per patient visit, like retinal practices, will fall at the high end of this collection per FTE per year range. Such practices may even generate up to $2 million in annual collections per insurance clerk. Elective practices (LASIK, elective plastics) and practices with a strong bias toward routine eye care have relatively little third-party billing to do, and can also get by with fewer patient accounts staff. Pediatric specialists will typically fall at the lower end of this range, with $800,000 in annual collections per clerk or less. Bread-and-butter general ophthalmology practices are at about $1 million annually per FTE, give or take.

Generally, these staff are all in-house. Of course, most practices typically outsource collections work on past-due accounts, and perhaps 10 percent of practices, especially smaller/solo practices, hire no in-house billing staff at all, and out-source billing duties to a local service firm. Such firms come in all sizes and levels of quality, from part-time freelancers running a small business on their kitchen table to large regional companies. The cost for the typical billing service ranges from 4 percent - 8 percent of collections. For mixed general and elective care practices, the large cash payments you collect in-house for services like LASIK and cosmetic plastic surgery should be charged at a lower rate or not included with you billing fees.

The advantages of hiring a competent outside billing service, especially for a small practice, are that they can deliver a higher level of expertise and greater cross-coverage. For example, if your small practice loses one key biller or coder or key computer operator, your cash flow could be interrupted for months. The chief disadvantages of an outside firm can be cost, dependency, and a loss of control.

Let's compare costs for a $1 million solo practice to stay in-house or go out of house for billing. Let's say our model practice finds a competent outside service at 6 percent of collections, a typical, even thrifty vendor, particularly in any urban setting. That's $60,000 per year. How does this stack up against doing the work in-house? Let's go down the list. Unless you've planned ahead, you're not going to save any facility costs (although you may be able to get an extra exam room or doctor's office out of the arrangement; if so, you should factor this in.).

As we've already covered, the typical $1 million practice will have one FTE devoted to the full range of patient accounts work. With outsourcing, that same practice will still have some residual in-house staff work to perform with a billing service engaged, even if it's just to traffic the super bills and other paperwork back and forth. Let's say you save 80 percent of one FTE, which, fully-burdened with benefits and taxes might run roughly $38,000—that comes to about $30,000 per year. You may also have computer savings of up to $20,000 per year (amortizing the typical system in place today, and keeping in mind that you'll still need in-house terminals for scheduling and to check patient balances.) So you are going to save about $50,000, but pay out about $60,000. In this scenario, it costs 20 percent more to outsource.

From this, you can see why the vast majority of practices handle their patient accounts work in-house. Let's assume your practice will, too. What kind of staff do you need? Put simply, you'll need clerks and a supervisor. Ideally, they'll be cross-trained enough to all know how to perform all of the objective tasks.

Department supervisors should be "working managers" in all but the largest settings. Here's a sample position description for the patient accounts department supervisor of a typical 3-5 doctor practice. Please note that in a smaller setting, the office manager is commonly responsible for all of these areas, plus management of the overall enterprise. Also note that we're describing here a combined department, inclusive of reception and patient accounts. More on this later.

POSITION DESCRIPTION

Patient Accounts and Reception Manager

Salary Range: Commensurate with experience, with up to a 10 percent discretionary annual performance bonus (The typical base salary range for suburban practices is $30,000 to $42,000 per year, which may go much higher than this in larger practices and urban clinics.)

Reports To: Administrator

Core Skills/Experience Inventory:

- Two or more years of experience supervising the reception and patient accounts function in a $3+ million medical practice, with an emphasis on serving Medicare beneficiaries (e.g.: ophthalmology, cardiology, orthopedics, etc.).
- The ability to step in and operate immediately; this is not a "learn on the job" setting or a manager trainee position, but one calling for a seasoned individual.
- The department manager must have a core competency in patient accounts management and have sufficient experience to become the internal key operator for the practice's computer system.
- This is a "working manager" position; the new manager must have sufficient working knowledge of the details of patient accounts to be able to post charges, submit claims, post payments, file secondary claims, challenge claim denials, and execute collection procedures. She/he should be able to sit in any chair of the department and perform the job functions of that person. (A side note here. Just as a doctor knows how to competently perform all of the job duties of a technician.)
- The supervisor must be able to establish and write down reasonable performance standards for each of these areas, train staff to these standards, and monitor ongoing performance.
- At least basic working knowledge of Microsoft Word and Excel.
- An undergraduate college education is preferred, but the level of formal education is secondary to real-world experience.
- Financial acumen sufficient to plan and manage to agreed departmental budgets and defined volume performance targets.
- A demonstrated ability to build and lead a staff team, and to actively mentor staff; rudimentary knowledge of employment law.

- The ability to communicate directly and clearly, in writing and speech.
- An extreme attention to operational detail and smooth daily operations in a complex and changing environment.
- The ability to contribute to the practice's business planning process.

Core Duties:

Broad Charter...Works with the administrator, practice owners and fellow employees to build and manage an economically successful, cohesive, high quality practice in our regional market.

- Reporting and Forecasting...Coordinates, with the administrator and practice accounting resources to periodically prepare various practice reports. Prepares the daily, weekly, and monthly computer system reports. Reviews the aged trial balance report monthly with the practice administrator and managing partner. Prepares and helps interpret monthly graphs showing over time the accounts receivable ratio and other key performance indices.
- Work Flow Engineering...With the administrator, works to develop and continuously fine-tune the complex flow of events, from the entry of patient demographics and marking of a super bill, through claims submission, tracking and payment.
- Doctor/Technician Education...Works with providers and clinical staff to assure that the superbill is consistently and accurately filled out; with the practice's administrator and managing partner, works to help reform the lagging compliance in this area of any providers.
- Front Desk Supervision...Supervises, through a designated "team leader," the work performance of the reception staff. Maintains a "quality improvement feedback loop" so that errors generated by the front desk and subsequently discovered by the insurance staff are brought to the attention of front desk.
- Performance Review and Enhancement...Develops volume performance goals (in terms of the A/R ratio, revenue and claims processed per clerk per year, etc.) and directs the resources required to meet these goals. Intervenes briskly if performance lags agreed levels.
- Committee Positions...Member of the Practice Management Committee composed of all supervisors, the administrator and the managing partner.
- Payer Relations...Maintains ongoing contacts with representatives of all of the practice's current and potential payers to assure that the practice's current

payments are aligned with contractual allowances and to facilitate periodic contracting efforts with potential payers.

- Supervisory and Recruitment Authority...Directly supervises, evaluates, and rewards/reprimands the work product of all staff in the department; in consultation with the administrator, has hiring and termination authority over all such staff. Involved in staff recruitment activities for the overall practice.

- Spending Authority...Has full on-budget spending authority; subject to review and oversight, has off-budget discretionary spending authority up to the limit of $150 total impact before consulting with the administrator. This spending authority will be subject to ongoing adjustment.

- Operations Documentation...Coordinates the preparation, maintenance and periodic revisions of the patient accounts section of the practice's operations manual; participates in the periodic review of the practice's staff policy manual.

The rest of the staff in the billing department might have a position description that looks like this:

POSITION DESCRIPTION
Patient Accounts Clerk

Salary Range: Commensurate with experience

Reports To: Patient Accounts and Reception Manager

Core Skills/Experience Inventory:

- One or more years of experience performing patient accounts function in a medical practice, with an emphasis on serving Medicare beneficiaries (e.g., ophthalmology, cardiology, orthopedics, etc.)

- Basic bookkeeping, phone and interpersonal skills; computer skills.

- Education: High school; college degree work is helpful but not required.

- The ability to step in and work immediately; this is not a trainee position, but one calling for a seasoned individual.

- Must have a diverse working knowledge of all details of patient accounts work and be able to post charges, submit claims, post payments, file secondaries, challenge claim denials and execute collection procedures.

- Ideally, prior experience with ______________, our computer system.
- The ability to communicate directly and clearly, in writing and verbally.
- The ability to contribute as a member of the overall practice team.

Duties:

[Note: Our practice seeks a patient account department with the highest possible level of cross-training among staff. This helps us cover vacations, share the workloads, and maintain skills redundancy. Therefore, all members of the department are ideally able to perform in all of the areas below. At any one time, you are likely to have a narrower list of core duties.]

- Participate in all staff meetings.
- Answer patient and payer questions over the phone.
- Know and periodically update the written provider guidelines from all payers.
- Review and audit patient charts and completed super bills for errors and omissions; know the correct coding and documentation standards for all practice services.
- Work with pre-approval/pre-certification/pre-determination/referrals, where required.
- Substitute for reception staff.
- Daily posting of charges (unless this is handled at the front desk).
- Daily submission of claims (paper and electronic).
- Prepare/mail patient statements.
- Follow up with payers on rejected claims and to check claims status.
- Sort/distribute incoming mail; open payments.
- Post payments and prepare deposits each day.
- Follow returned check protocol.
- Prepare daily and monthly period closings and reconciliations.
- Participate in the generation and review of various daily, weekly and monthly computer system reports, including the monthly aged trial balance reports.
- Continuously and persistently learn from your errors, which, given the complexity of this area of the practice, may initially be very frequent.
- Work with older accounts and make recommendations for accounts to be turned over to collections.

- Monitor trends in payments and denials and inform the department heads of these trends.
- Maintain cordial relationships with all payer representatives.
- Prepare refunds.
- Participate with the preparation and periodic revisions of the patient accounts section of the practice's operations manual.
- Any other duties that may be required in any department for smooth operation of the practice.

The rest of the staff on the reception side of the overall department might have a position description that looks like this:

POSITION DESCRIPTION
Front Desk Clerk / Receptionist

Salary Range: Commensurate with experience

Reports To: Patient Accounts and Reception Manager, or the reception desk "Team Leader"

Core Skills/Experience Inventory:

- One or more years of experience performing reception functions in a medical practice.
- Basic phone and interpersonal skills; computer skills.
- Able to interact with patients in a pleasant, efficient and professional manner; resistant to the periodic stresses of the front desk and able to cheerfully assist complaining patients.
- Education: High school; college degree or work is helpful but not required.
- This may be a trainee/entry position, or one calling for a seasoned individual, depending on practice preference and the local job market.
- Ideally, prior experience with _______________, our computer system.
- The ability to communicate directly and clearly, in writing and verbally.
- The ability to contribute as a member of the overall practice team.

Duties:

[Note: Our practice seeks a reception and patient accounts department with the highest possible level of cross-training among staff. This helps us cover vacations, share the work loads, and maintain skills redundancy. Therefore, all members of the department are ideally able to eventually perform in all of the areas below. At any one time, you are likely to have a narrower list of core duties.]

- Participate in all staff meetings.
- Answer and route calls from patients, vendors, payers and other providers.
- Check patients in and out of the practice.
- Inspect and tidy the reception and other public areas of the practice periodically.
- Be on the lookout for distressed or unhappy patients, and help them resolve their issues.
- Know and help to periodically update the written provider guidelines from all payers.
- Work with patient account staff to audit patient charts and super bills for errors and omissions; know the correct coding and documentation standards for all practice services.
- Continuously and persistently learn from your errors which, given the complexity of this area of the practice, may initially be very frequent
- Assist with pre-approval/pre-certification/pre-determination/referrals, where required.
- Substitute for billing and collections staff.
- Post daily charges (unless this is batched and handled by the billing staff).
- Help prepare patient statements
- Help to sort/distribute incoming mail; open payments.
- Participate in the generation and review of various daily, weekly and monthly computer system reports, including the monthly aged trial balance reports.
- Monitor trends in patient responses to various office policies and report these to the department head.
- Participate with the preparation and periodic revisions of the reception section of the practice's operations manual.
- Any other duties that may be required in any department for smooth operation of the practice.

How and where can you find these paragons of staffing excellence? In a word, you are often best off *raiding* them from other well-run practices, unless your practice is so large that you can afford to have a few green staff at the bottom of the ladder in training positions. This area of the practice is not like practice marketing, or even technical work, where there may be several acceptable ways to do the job well. Unfortunately, there is only one right way to do most of the above jobs, especially in billing, where there are hundreds of incorrect ways to post charges, submit claims, and get paid for the work that you all do. Some of these errors can be catastrophically damaging to your practice's cash flow.

Beyond the usual classified ads and calls to placement agencies, it may make sense to:

- Develop a close relationship with your computer vendor to help you network with other users in your area. It's a huge advantage to bring in staff who are already familiar with your system;
- If necessary, hire an outside agent to call or visit other well-run practices in the region, ask for the billing department, and offer a finder's fee for information leading to a hire. [Simultaneously, make sure that your own staff are paid and treated well enough to be immune from such poaching by other practices!];
- Make sure you hire from the top, downward. There's no sense loading up your department with people who don't entirely know their jobs, with no real guru, and end up with the blind leading the blind. On the other hand, hiring a truly superior supervisor and building on their strength is a wonderful formula for success; and
- Make sure that you have enough staff on board. If you've allowed the billing department to get behind (as, for example, when the >90 days accounts exceed about 18 percent of total receivables), you will need additional staff, at least temporarily, to keep up. A practice that's growing 10 percent a year should have a billing department that is mildly over-staffed enough so it doesn't feel hard-pressed and is ready to easily absorb the growing claims volume. Conversely, a practice that's shrinking (losing doctors, closing down satellite offices) should be proportionately downsizing the billing staff to keep costs in line.

Let's cover additional success factors of superior reception and patient accounts management. Administrators often ask, "Should we divide up our billing work alphabetically or by payer?" With small practices that only employ one or two billing staff, everyone obviously has to do everything (and NO practice should have just one person who knows the patient accounts routine. In the smallest solo practice, the office manager will commonly handle billing, but the doctor needs to know how to post charges and submit claims, as well, just as a backup.).

With somewhat larger billing teams, it makes good sense to divide accounts up alphabetically, so that you are not vulnerable to the departure of a single key employee. With extremely large practices, let's say those over $12 million in annual collections, an argument can be made for having the billing staff become more specialized. However, you should make sure that cross-training is sufficient and that key payers (Medicare, the Blues, etc.) can be handled by at least two resident staff experts.

We should also cover proper office facilities for your patient accounts staff, although this may seem trivial at first glance. The proper husbandry, care, and feeding of these key employees is critical. Think about the nature of this work: It's very precise, very dull, and can be maddeningly elaborate. It's easy to get distracted and lose your place. You have to be able to hear people on the telephone. Just because they have little direct contact with the public doesn't mean insurance clerks should work in the basement.

The worst possible setting is to put your insurance staff, almost as an afterthought, in a hallway—this is much too commonly done. The result is constant interruption by passing staff, high error rates and very low output. The ideal arrangement is a large/airy room and cubicles for every staff member. The partitioning walls should be fabric-covered for soundproofing, and about five feet high—tall enough to block out the world when you are sitting, but low enough for most staff to peer over if they have a question for their neighbor, or just need a little human contact.

Ideally, there are windows in the room, and the positions of the cubicles give most staff a glimpse of the outside world. But watch out for too much light, which will increase the strain of looking at a computer screen all day. In terms of economic priority, the efficiency and quality of the workspace for your billing staff falls secondary only to the workspace for your doctors. It's your *cash flow*, after all.

Growth and development of a practice can cause even the best-run business office to wobble. As the practice balloons, diligent reception, and billing staff can bite their lip and absorb ever-more work, resulting in burnout and a precipitous climb in both errors and payment delays. Even small, simple, solo practices have lots of moving parts. This enterprise complexity grows logarithmically with scale. Your reception/patient accounts manager should have a prominent voice in business planning meetings and help you forecast the team's breaking point. Make sure you're staying in that zone of plus-or-minus $1 million in annual collections per billing FTE.

Right-sizing the reception staff is more a matter of your individual practice flow, patient mix, the efficiency of the involved staff members, and the level of service and hand-holding you want your patients to experience. As an internal exercise, once you get the ratio about right, divide your daily patient visits by the number of receptionists, and you'll go forward with a ratio that fits your unique setting.

Remember that it's always false economy to skimp on clerical staff, whose duties include recall and continuity of care. Such staff need enough time to think up a appropriate comeback to a patient who doesn't want to pay that day, instead of just letting them walk out the door for free. Such staff need to be rested enough to be able to chat for a minute with a patient who is considering surgery. There MUST be enough time and staff coverage to call no-shows, update charts, and enter long-range appointment times (instead of taking the easy way out and simply sending a recall card.)

Reception staff have to be in sufficient abundance to allow for training time, and to allow everyone to have heads clear enough to remember where to look to see if Mrs. Ratner's payer requires her to have a referral before her office visit. And they have to be able to explain in absolutely convincing terms to a suspicious, oppositional octogenarian and her daughter why a refraction fee has to be collected, even if she isn't buying glasses until next week.

The pressure on receptionists is even higher in those practices where check out staff are expected to post charges. Admittedly, posting at checkout is ideal: If you know how to post a charge, odds go up that you know what kind of co-payment or deductible to collect. But empirically, unless you have just the right people in place, it's difficult for a high-traffic check out clerk to simultaneously (and accurately) post charges. That's why in a majority of practices we still recommend batch posting of charges by staff who work behind the scenes, whether you have one office or a string of satellites. The only exception is in those practices that have gone through a slow, deliberate and successful process to develop front desk staff that can multi-task.

Reception staff get into trouble from all angles. They get into trouble with patients that ask when they will be seen, because, "The doctor is now 17 minutes behind!" They get into trouble with vendors, who wonder why they can't help make the patient waiting time even worse by letting the salesman in to see the doctor on a busy clinic day. They get glares from technicians, who feel overworked. They get disparaging memos from their colleagues in billing who are peeved about one transposed address out of 300 entries. Finally, they get harassment from doctors, who feel over-scheduled at 51 patients, and under-scheduled at 49 patients. On top of all that, the doctors rarely come up to the front desk with anything nicer than a reproach, even IF precisely *50* patients are scheduled that day. If your practice has superior receptionists, give them money and prizes and praise before your competition, reading this same chapter, takes them off your hands.

Well-meaning efforts to modernize, economize, and reduce the stresses and labor demands of the reception area often go awry. With rising costs, it's common for practices to resort to caller-prompted automatic routing. Avoid this if possible. In addition, resorting to the perceived economy of automated appointment reminder calls has a rebound effect. Our experience in the field is that practices using automated calling for appointment reminders have their no-show rates increase 50 percent to 100 percent.

In the billing department, there are similar do's and don'ts gained from years in the field with highly successful clients.

Great billing requires very unusual kinds of people. They need to be smart enough to master the labyrinth of billing, obsessed enough to want to get their work perfected, and possess a high enough boredom threshold to stay at the job some 2000 hours a year. Art majors need not apply, in most cases. Nor are most extroverts happy for very long cavorting with figures more than people all day long. Burnout is rampant, without some thoughtful care and feeding. This should include:

- Liberal meeting and education time…the constantly changing environment demands it;
- A high level of job flexibility…fortunately, not all of a billing clerk's hours have to be mainstreamed with the rest of the staff. Sometimes the early hours of the morning are a perfect time to catch up, and this also allows staff to be with their kids after school. At the other end of the clock, evening hours can allow staff to work open patient-responsible accounts (which, of course, should have been largely collected at the time of service.); and
- Superior supervision…this supervision is best done by an experienced biller. In settings where the general bookkeeper or other person without billing experience supervises the department, morale and productivity can be low.

Written protocols are another major billing department success factor. These need frequent updating, and should form the core of your training program. Protocols should be in sufficient detail to outline specific keystrokes needed to accomplish various tasks. For example:

"To prepare an aging report, select 'Menu 8,' 'option #2.' Enter the desired fields according to the screen's prompts. Enter 'print.' This will print a report with outstanding balances for all patients by payer…."

Your procedure manual should be sure to include daily, weekly, and monthly checklists, which can also be extremely helpful. Even the best-trained pilots resort to written checklists without embarrassment before they take off. And flying the billing department of a modern ophthalmic clinic is vastly more complex than flying a Cessna.

The major secondary gain of checklists, from the perspective of the department manager and administrator, is that it vastly reduces the supervision time. Relevant staff, each with their own checklist to mark up and turn in, can more readily be left to their own self-supervision, with less frequent hovering and oversight.

<u>Sample Daily Checklist Items:</u>

- ❑ Did we post the day's charges by day's end?
- ❑ Did we submit electronically?
- ❑ Did the clinic run on time today?
- ❑ Have the next day's patients been called?
- ❑ Were all of today's no-shows called?

Sample Weekly Checklist Items:

- ❑ Have timecards been entered and payroll called in?
- ❑ Was an office supplies run made?
- ❑ Have this week's recall card's been mailed?
- ❑ Have caller logs been forwarded to marketing for tabulation?

<u>Sample Monthly Checklist Items:</u>

- ❑ Has the month been closed at the same time for both the patient accounts system and the general ledger?
- ❑ Has the appointment template been advanced another month?
- ❑ Are all of the end of the month reports printed and bound?
- ❑ Has the aged trial balance report been reviewed with the doctor?

Checklists like this will keep important—but not urgent—items in your plain view. It's easy in small, harried departments to have a month slip by and forget to generate the month-ending aging report because you're full-up with other duties.

How about for those difficult patients who refuse to pay their patient-responsible/self-pay amounts? First, you need to have the doctors' permission to pursue deadbeats. You probably already have escalating dunning letters, leading to, "If this account is not paid or suitable payment arrangements made within the next 10 days your account will be referred to an outside agency for collections." Obviously, the longer you delay vigorous internal action, or sending patients to a collection agency, the lower your chances go for financial recovery. Warmer hearts are chilling as the economy softens and overall fees decline. If your doctor has been reticent to send patients to a collection agency in the past, ask again. At the very least, try one last annual shot at laggard patients with a year-end offer of amnesty from further pursuit if they'll write a check for 50 percent to 80 percent of their outstanding bill by the end of the year.

Simple human error, often starting first at the front desk, is the bane of every insurance clerk. Some of these clerks and their department heads hold their tongue and silently correct repeated front desk errors. This may help to keep the peace, but at a large cost in continued errors. It's much better to bring entry errors and other gaffs right back to the person who goofed and gently ask them to correct it personally. Their learning curve will accelerate, and billing staff frustrations will be reduced. The same approach goes, obviously, if the problem starts with doctors or technical staff. Always bring the error back to its source for correction.

The grossest kind of clinic floor errors lead to missing superbills, which should be traced at the end of every day with a missing ticket or unclosed encounter report. More commonly, scribes and providers simply forget to check off boxes. In the typical setting, $3 to $10 on average is dropped from the average patient visit....not much money when you think about a single patient. But this adds up to tens of thousands of dollars over the course of a year. You simply have to sweat the details.

Given what's at stake, and the complexities of coding, most advisors these days like to put the responsibility back on the doctors—and not the scribes—to fill out the superbill. As a backup, there should be at least one lay person in the practice who works themselves into the position of the company's guru and troubleshooter. This person should supervise regular audits, training and manual writing, and is most commonly the head of billing or the practice administrator or even a dedicated specialist who also handles the compliance program in larger practices.

Make sure that you are matching departmental resources to departmental standards. It would be unfair to task your billing staff with an exceptionally high level of reporting and oversight, while giving them an exceptionally low level of resources (staff, facilities, equipment, training, PRN overtime, etc.) Remember through all of this that the administrator is the *resource allocation authority* who needs to balance practice standards (as articulated by the board) with practical economic matters.

Too often, departments are too segregated from each other in practices and live in their own boxes. The technical staff never really develop an appreciation for the challenges in billing and vice-versa. This leads to the development of competitive factions. You can break this down by exposing every new staff member to each area of the practice—allowing a slated front desk clerk, for example, to see surgery, and observe patient encounters for a morning. Once they better understand the "product" you sell, they'll do a much better job representing your services to the public *and helping you get paid for these valuable services.*

One problem we often see is that billing department goals are too diffuse and amount to little more than, "You all try your best, and let's see how much we can bring in this month." It's far more effective to set specific goals. Examples are an agreed date in the calendar by which time total accounts receivable fall below an agreed figure. Or a target for your accounts receivable ratio (A/R divided by average charges.) It's especially helpful to designate the percentage of total A/R that should be out past 90-days, typically 18 percent or less is the performance target. In Chapter Ten we cover a host of appropriate benchmarks, which—if your reception and patient accounts staff are appropriately organized—should be easy to hit.

How can you detect if your patient accounts team falls behind? There are several signals. Seek out staff that are in the middle of posting charges or submitting claims to tell you what date the service was performed. If the answer is over 72 hours ago, someone has fallen behind. Examine the frequency of patient refund checks—it should be monthly. Ask staff where they keep their rejected claims, and examine the file. A large collection of unworked rejections is a common sign of getting behind. Look at the aged trial balance (aging) report and ask at random for the status of larger/old open accounts. If staff don't know the status of most such accounts by rote, they may be falling behind.

There are many effective sources for help with billing department problems. All serve a purpose. You can turn to your computer vendor. You can call on local and national billing consultants. One of the most overlooked resources are the staff in other eye care practices just like yours. You and your colleague may compete vigorously for cataract cases, but it's very useful to develop relationships between patient accounts departments. It may even be helpful to pull together formal site visits among collaborating practices and to hold periodic group meetings to compare billing notes.

At this point, we rather expect that you and other fellow readers may be exhausted. With so much to learn to run even a modest practice, and so much to try to get done—precisely right—all at the same time, what are the odds of success? The frank answer is that the odds of your practice achieving perfection are very low. Even in the most scrupulous settings, excessive charges are added and neglected charges are dropped. There is no way around the fact that patient accounts work is mind-numbingly dull. So how can we get doctors, techs, and others in the practice who need to know coding and reimbursement details cold up to speed? While some advisors focus on the negative, and point out all of the adverse consequences of error, we like to concentrate on the positive results of getting it right: Peace of mind. Maximum compensation. A sense of mastery and control. There are no problems, just opportunities.

In summary, here are ten top "rules," success factors for your reception and patient accounts management department

1. Make sure you have enough of the right staff to get the job done properly.
2. Make sure you have sufficient cross-coverage and cross-training to never have just one person who knows a critical job, no matter how small the practice.
3. Develop, update, and refer often to clear, written protocols.
4. Make sure staff are trained with the use of written protocols.
5. The administrator and at least one doctor need to be highly conversant with your computer system and your billing protocols.
6. Use the written protocols to periodically inspect accuracy and efficiency.
7. Employ graphs over 12-24 month or longer periods to track trends in the collection ratio, A/R ratio, collections per billing department FTE per month, etc.

8. Visit successful reception and billing departments in other practices and copy all of the things that they do better than you.
9. Develop both internal and external sources of expertise for billing problems as they arise. A few dollars spent for expertise now can help you avoid under-billing, uncertainty and costly adverse audits.
10. Invest in at least bi-annual refresher training courses with your computer vendor.

Chapter Eight:

The Role of Providers, as Owners and as Workers, in Optimizing Cash Flow and Keeping the Company Alive

The year is 2141, ages and ages into the future. Based on current trends, we can nearly picture the ophthalmologist of that distant time. In profile, he (or she) looks more like a gymnast than a clinician. He's wearing a Lycra body suit, high-traction shoes, and a wireless ear piece and microphone that was implanted years earlier for convenience.

With a word or two into his microphone, "Dr. Lycra" can call up data on the next patient, including the provisional diagnosis and treatment plan, which have dropped out of a formula from all prior, automated workups and pre-testing. Around his waist, looking a little like a futuristic cop's crowded holster, is a tool belt, festooned with a hands-free indirect, an occluder (a sentimental antique from his great-great-grandfather's practice) and a solid-state, infinitely tunable, hand-held laser. On one hand, he wears a thin glove—an array of the most common drops and ointments can be delivered to his fingertips from a pouch at his side. During each exam, the practice's voice recognition software records the doctor's chart notes, and without being asked provides prompts for any missing data or overlooked questions. Annoying, but effective. And it's eliminated many malpractice suits.

After the exam, color-coded lights that seemingly float mid-air in the center of the hallway, direct patients to their next destination in the practice. "A pleasure seeing you this morning, Ms. Hays," says Dr. Lycra. "Based on our tests, that cataract in your left eye will be ready for laser extraction in about 38 or 39 months, we're not precisely sure yet. Please follow the green flashing light to Robby in optical. He already has your complete record going all the way back to 2041 when you were a little girl. He also has your new prescription and has picked out the 10 most popular frames in the North American Alliance for women with your beautiful skin coloring and bone structure. I know you're going to love what you see! It's amazing, really. You know we almost stopped selling glasses 40 years ago, until they became big fashion again. But listen to me talk. Here I am 72 and going on like a guy who's ready to retire. I'll see you right here in 37 months. You'll get our auto-notice, as always."

At 10:04am, just 26 minutes after she arrived in the clinic for a complete exam, Ms. Hays is back on the street. She only interacted with two real people, her doctor and her optician. The rest of the time, she simply followed the logical directions of one video screen and one gentle, disembodied voice after another. Meanwhile, in not much more time than it's taking you to read this paragraph, Dr. Lycra has seen another patient and squeezed in a few more seconds to push the button that rebalances his nutritional and energy state. He's all set for the last 47 patients of the morning before meeting his wife for lunch at noon. And just incidentally, he'll have to remove about three or four cataracts that afternoon to pay for lunch. Unless they order dessert, of course.

Unfortunately, we don't have a time machine. We can't come back here to the present early years of the 21st Century after a trip to the future, and bring back all of Dr. Lycra's labor-saving and energy-boosting devices. But we had better do something. And fast. Based on current trends in reimbursement, and the slowly rising cost of doing business, your personal income as a surgeon is destined to be falling year after year unless you are able to improve your personal productivity.

The math is rather simple. Let's say you see an average of 35 patients per day, 3½ days a week, 48 weeks a year, and have an average ticket of $150 per patient visit and run a practice with a 60 percent overhead. You'll make about $350,000 this year. With this common scenario, if there's a net fee reduction of just 5 percent, and all expenses stay the same, you'll be taking a 12 percent pay cut. If expenses also go up at a typical 3 percent, you'll take a 17 percent net pay cut.

To make up for these impacts, you would need to see about another 7 percent more patients, or 2½ patients per day. This productivity gain is a lot more likely to be accomplished than the 8 percent cost savings it would take to yield the same profit restoration. Getting rid of 8 percent of your costs in a single year would be equivalent to lopping off one full-time staff member in a solo practice, or nearly all of the marketing or facility costs. You simply can't keep that up year after year. The best, most practical, reasonably sustainable way to slay the fee reduction dragon is with increased personal productivity. And you don't need Dr. Lycra's slick suit or tool belt to get there.

The starting point is to first measure productivity for every doctor in your practice, and in every setting if you have multiple offices. There are numerous, meaningful ways to measure a doctor's productivity.

Weeks worked per year is the grossest measure of a doctor's output, and doesn't really count much except whether or not the doctor is showing up for work. Most physician and optometrist employment contracts specify the maximum allowable number of vacation days or weeks permitted…for partner-level doctors, this usually tops out at about 13 weeks or fewer off per year, before a partner has to revert to being an associate.

Hours worked per year, as a metric, is a bit more precise and constraining. We've seen doctors who didn't like being boxed into eight or ten weeks of vacation per year by their partners, so they started working six hours a day to get even. Anything north of 2000 hours a year is a reasonable target for a full-time doctor; hard-working practice owners often work more than 2500 hours per year.

How about patient visits per doctor per month? Now we're getting somewhere, and measuring more than attendance. We're looking at raw through-put. For an energetic general ophthalmologist, we like to coach clients toward not less than 550 patient visits per average month, admittedly somewhat higher than the average eye surgeon. If you see patients in clinic 3½ days per week, 3½ weeks in the typical month, that comes to about 45 patient visits per day or about one patient every 10 minutes, not counting breaks and other time off the clinic floor. Optometrists (and slower medical ophthalmologists, depending of course on the patient mix) should be able to see 300+ visits per month. Subspecialist ophthalmologists should fall between these two extremes, seeing somewhere in the range of 450 or more patient visits per month.

Patient flow within any given day should also be studied. Keep in mind that the process of measuring clinic flow in any kind of internal study like this will lead to everyone on the floor speeding up. Just seeing that they really *can* move faster is motivation enough for some clinic teams to see how much more efficient they can become. Below is a sample grid that you can use as-is or modify to gain insights into your own clinic bottlenecks.

PROVIDER TIME STUDY

Purpose: To gain insights into an individual physician's use of clinic time and to distinguish between inefficiencies that are staff/room/equipment related vs. doctor-behavior related.

Instructions: Select a typical clinic half-day. Select as unbiased an observer as possible. It may be useful to repeat the study on successive days with successive observers. Start from the time of the provider's arrival at the clinic. Enter a brief description of the doctor's activity, and shift to a new line with every material change in activity.

Date___________________

Total patient visits _________

Subject___________________

Observer__________________

Activity	Start Time	Stop Time	Total Time	Observations/Comments	Doctor Affability with Patient, Family, Staff
Example: *Visit with sales rep to discuss new viscoelastic*	*10:13a*	*10:35a*	*0:22*	*Clinic was already running 30 minutes behind when a drug rep arrived; all but the first 3 minutes of the sales call was social time talking about sports cars.*	*N/A*

Used in combination with a more traditional time study in the clinic, where each *patient's* start and stop time is measured at each station, this *doctor* time study can identify gaps in the doctor's concentration and demonstrate the corrosive effects of late arrival, dawdling, taking personal phone calls, and similar sins on cash flow.

You can take this process engineering to amazing lengths, and with willing doctors markedly increase their throughput without any appreciable wear and tear on the "machinery."

Of course, clinic time and volume is just one piece of the equation. Under many fee schedules, the cost to transit a patient is barely covered by the basic exam fee. In most practices, all meaningful net cash flow stems from surgical procedures and optical sales. Try dividing the number of patient visits you see in a month by the number of cataract, Lasik and other major surgical cases. Unless you have a young practice, an especially conservative practice, or work in a competitive market, the result should ideally be a number at or under 25, that's to say, you should see about 25 patients or fewer before coming across each surgical case (defining "case" as a single eye.). If you dispense, the optical density of your practice should mean that you sell about $200 in optical goods for every $1,000 in professional medical/surgical services you sell (omitting ASC fees, but including special testing fees). If your surgical and optical densities are well off these norms, you may have a great opportunity for profit improvement.

Next, divide your annual collections by the total number of patients you see in a year (including un-paid post-op visits.) If you're the typical doctor, this "average ticket" number should come close to $150. It will be some $15 to $30 or more higher if you dispense glasses and MUCH higher if you include collections from a surgical center. It might be lower than $150 if you're surgically conservative, or are constrained by a managed-care heavy market or a setting with an excess number of providers for the population base.

In at least purely commercial if not especially professional-sounding terms, "profit per doctor hour" is the gold standard for seeing how your productivity measures up against your peers. Simply take the total annual profits before depreciation and doctor compensation (including salary, draws, officer entitlements, perks, etc.) and divide this profit figure by the number of hours your doctor/s worked in the same year. The number may be as low as $60, or as high as $600 or more. What counts in not so much how you stack up against your peers, of course, inside or outside your practice, but how you're doing compared to yourself in each successive year of your career. As an aside, this is a great way to determine if your satellite office work is worth the time, trouble, and travel compared to your main office.

Patient satisfaction counts, too, of course. Raw productivity, without both the perception and reality of great caring, is a prescription for practice disaster. If you've recently turned up the heat, and are now more highly productive in raw patient visit terms—but in your hurrying convey a sense of disregard or indifference—you're just going to do harm to your practice all the faster, not help the bottom line.

The most productive surgeons we know move through their clinic with an economy of motion, a sort of ophthalmic ballet, that's probably as hard to master as the real thing. If you can't work more elegantly, you'll have to settle for longer hours and greater intensity, and thrash along as best you can. You'll have to avoid as many wasted steps as possible, stay on the clinic floor, and stay off the phone as much as possible. Save your Internet and e-mail time for the end of the day. You should be arriving somewhat before the first patients, and huddle with technical staff about the day ahead, and then start the clinic alongside them, helping them work up the first few post-ops and quick checks.

If you find yourself mentally foggy at the end of a day of patients, you're doing something wrong. Get more sleep. Take a noon nap of not less than 20 minutes. (This is an old trick courtesy of the U.S. Navy Seals...anything less this will not work against any sleep debt, and may actually leave you groggier than you started.) Eat better (more protein, fewer carbohydrates seems to help many), smaller and more frequent meals. Exercise. If appropriate, take off those extra few pounds and inches—imagine how much more energy you would have at the end of the day if you didn't have those extra 20 pounds hanging around.

What else is under the doctor's control to help augment cash flow? The opportunities are nearly endless. If you're like the average mid-career or older surgeon that we meet with, you may need to diversify your service mix and put more "products" on your practice "shelf." If you are imprinted solely to cataracts you may be blind to the other services you could be offering patients. It's a useful exercise to pull each doctor's charge reports for a year, and to compare this to payer-supplied benchmarks. Dry eye treatment, retinoscopy, and visual field exams are often underutilized. Even within your multi-doctor clinic, you may find vast differences between providers in their mix of services. A group discussion about this finding may lead to not only opportunities for individual improvement, but for increased internal cross-referral.

In a multi-physician practice, it may also be very revealing to look at the collection ratio and A/R ratio of each doctor. Of course, there will be an expected variance based on practice patterns and patient mix. But for two general ophthalmologists/cataract surgeons in the same practice, the collection ratio should be essentially the same. Look for both the obvious and the subtle disparities. Is one doctor the sole contractor for a low-paying contract? Or does one doctor's behaviors (like hoarding charts after surgery and not dictating or coding the case for several weeks) explain the difference?

Make sure you're thinking not just about payer-allowed procedures, but elective care. On what portion of your cataract surgical patients do you perform intraoperative or postoperative relaxing incisions for astigmatism? Although new lens materials and smaller incisions have markedly reduced induced astigmatism, thousands of patients go to cataract surgery every year with pre-existing astigmatism, and are never asked by their doctors if they would like this corrected for a reasonable fee. Do you have hand mirrors in every exam room? Handing a mirror to patients with droopy lids that are not yet functionally but are certainly cosmetically candidates for surgery, and then standing behind them to demonstrate what blepharoplasty could do for them, is remarkably effective.

Affable doctors generally make a better income than grouches Many ophthalmologists could use at least a little bit of help in their rapport with patients. If you genuinely want to get better in this area, formal videotaped coaching may be able to help. On the other hand, if you feel that you can't make further reforms in this area, try to delegate every conceivable moment of your face-to-face time to ODs and tech extenders. This will anger those patients who would like to develop a warm relationship with their surgeon, and some may leave, but this approach will, on balance, result in a better experience for patients if you are truly an incurable grump.

On the flip side of the coin, don't go too far to the side of being Dr. Nice-Guy. Don't give away an excessive amount of courtesy services because this leads to two problems: First, it can demoralize your staff (especially if on the same day you're ranting about cash flow); and second, taken too far, it can displace paying patients. We remember one popular client in a small town who gave services away to nearly 5 percent of his patients. There are less expensive ways to cement friendships. This same misplaced generosity applies to keeping refraction fees below market rates. Some clinics still charge a $10 nuisance fee; these days, they should be in the $20+ range. Similarly, don't allow optical customers to receive their glasses before paying half-down when they order and in full at the time of pickup.

At the end of the exam, even if you have a scribe in the room, it's important to your cash flow to be heads-up and deeply engaged with what gets entered on the superbill. Doctors are in the best position to know what has just been done for their patient, and they generally have more intellectual horsepower than anyone in the building. They have the most at stake for coding an exam correctly, both to optimize reimbursement and to avoid fraudulent billing. Our suggestion is that the doctor personally fills out the superbill, or alternately dictates it, and then reviews with more than a glance what has been entered.

Of course, doctors both aid and detract from cash flow in ways that extend well beyond the clinic floor. It's essential in our view that doctor-owners become conversant with their computer systems and at least the general details of patient accounts flow and business operations in the practice. The more geographically remote the practice, the more important these skills become—because it's all that much harder to find experienced staff should you lose a key office manager or biller. It's essential that as a practice owner you not only have access to the numbers, and the operational details, but that you understand them.

Here's an apocryphal example, but typical when we audit a practice for the first time. The doctor will say, "We have a splendid recall system. I always nominate a return-to-clinic order and the staff always enters it." The office manager will say,

"We have a great recall system. We send out cards, and most of our patients come back on time." The clerical staff will then say, "We have a pretty-good recall system. We send out cards whenever we have the time. Anytime one of our cards get sent back with a bad address, we try to call the patient." Finally, we go to the stacks of charts. And the two-year and older charts say to us, "Thanks for stopping by. We've been sitting up here on the shelf gathering dust. Nobody bothers to open us up and find out what happened to our owners, the patients. Will somebody please give them a call?"

Surely, there could be few elements of running a practice more fundamental than regular financial statements and a solid recall system, yet these basics are absent in a remarkable number of otherwise fine, high-quality organizations, largely because the doctors in the practice don't demand it.

After you've mastered the small details, it's also essential to know the big picture. You should know the sum of all of the parts of your business, especially when the business has been subdivided into divisions to keep the accounting straight or to partition off liability. On top of this, you need to be well-advised on your personal financial plan, so you can truly see the big, consolidated picture. Decisions you make about investing in your business will have an influence on your at-home cash flow, and vice-versa.

This week hundreds, perhaps thousands of fresh, new business ideas will noisily spring to life in America, rosy cheeked, fully funded, their CEOs charging hard toward dreams of wild success. In the very same week, about the same number of businesses will be smothered, voluntarily or otherwise. Off to oblivion.

Obviously, the vast majority of you reading this are working in enterprises that fall somewhere between these two extremes of nascence and demise. The happy truth is that eye care is an extremely difficult business to wreck. You have to really, really work hard to go completely out of business as an eye surgeon. That doesn't keep some ophthalmologists from trying, however. Here are the most frequent cliffhangers we run into:

- "I'll just slow my practice down a little and keep my hand in for a few more years part-time." Ophthalmology is a largely fixed-cost business. At 40 percent net profit margins, a 25 percent drop in production results in up to a 60% collapse in profits.
- "Sure, I've got more than my share of malpractice cases, but that's because I live in a city with hungry lawyers." Unless you're a hyper-volume LASIK surgeon,

more than one or two malpractice cases in your career should be a warning to stop and solve whatever it is that's the problem. Nine times out of ten, it's not a frank clinical problem, so much as a problem with patient relationships.

- "We need more surgical cases. Let's just ramp up our advertising." Advertising is like pain medicine: Necessary and highly helpful when used in the right doses, addictive when used inappropriately. And it can mask other practice problems. Spending more than 5 percent of revenue for marketing in the typical general practice or 10 percent in a LASIK practice long-term may be a sign that something is awry with the underlying organization.
- "I don't need disability insurance. I'm in great shape, and besides, if I'm out for a couple of months, the practice could carry on without me." Could it really? Run the numbers, consult a reputable insurance broker, decide if you're under-insured, and act accordingly.
- "I don't need an attorney to advise me on this contract. It's pretty straight forward." We continue to be amazed at how many surgeons making seven-figure incomes begrudge their attorneys, accountants, and other advisors a few thousand tax-deductible dollars a year to keep them out of trouble.
- "I know we can't really afford it right now, but I'd really like to buy a ________." You fill in the blank. It could be a new office complex or a cutting edge piece of equipment. Any purchase that exceeds 5 percent of your annual collections that is not absolutely required to meet clinical quality assurance requirements should be subjected to formal economic analysis for a reasonable payback period or return on investment. This includes most newly posted staff positions.

When you've scanned the business headlines in recent years and seen the Enron, Global Crossings, and other stark news break , you probably thought to yourself, "There's not much for me to learn from this." Think again. Business is business. And all businesses are fragile, living creatures. Somebody has to be their guardians, stewards and watchdogs. Your ophthalmology business, while less fragile than the weakest of Wall Street's wobbling giants, needs your daily care, vigilance, and feeding.

Beyond issues of raw clinical productivity, we also need to address the more subjective issue of doctor-doctor and doctor-administrator interactions. Once upon a time, physician leadership had little influence on ophthalmic economic success. Until ten years ago, few practices faced any real commercial adversity. Allowable fees were high. General ophthalmology was a tidy bundle of largely geriatric services delivered in mostly solo practices. Patients were plentiful and operating costs were comparatively low.

However, an increasing number of practices are sputtering today. Why? The core reason is that physician leadership skills are still trying to catch up with the blistering pace of change in the business of medicine.

Although most new clients believe they are harmed by culprits called "managed care," or "competition," they are most often in trouble because they have not scaled up the time and quality of their leadership to match the growing size and complexity of their organizations. This is intensified in practices growing rapidly through consolidation. It's due to these changes that the management skills of your practice's lead physician will have more impact on your success over the next ten years than any other single factor. Wise choices are critical, even if that boils down to who's going to be the managing partner of a two-doctor practice.

Practice leaders are most often selected because they are the oldest or most financially productive doctors. This does not always correlate with leadership skills. In non-medical business settings, the most profitable use of an owner's time is often management. Not so in ophthalmology, where time spent on the clinic floor and in the O.R. is the most profitable, especially because few group practices pay their lead partners a management stipend, and compensation is commonly indexed to individual production. Pick a leader in your practice whose skill and time commitment matches the unique challenges in your particular setting. Then give them their area to run with enough responsibility, authority, and accountability to the other doctors in the group.

One of the greatest financial impacts on practices, for better or worse, is the way that partners interact in a practice. Benjamin Franklin once famously said: "Keep your eyes wide open before marriage, and half shut afterwards." He could have just as readily been giving advice to partnering eye surgeons, who today have a disharmony and divorce rate that nearly matches that of the ordinary kind of matrimony.

Even in the most congenial practices we visit, significant time has to be spent getting at least one or two strained relationships back on track. Through the years we've developed a simple how-to list of recommendations that may help you reverse partner discord, or, even better, stay out of trouble in the first place.

<u>Partnership Rules</u>

1. Don't compare your "deal" (your hours, wage, call schedule, case mix, burden of scutt work, etc.) with those of your partners and get burned up because Joe gets more cataracts than you get, or Mary earns more than you do, or the practice's

senior partner is now off call rotation. Instead, it's a lot easier on your nerves to compare your present situation as a partner with what life would be like as a soloist. We often counsel junior partners who are steamed because they don't have the same high surgical loads or incomes as the senior doctors, "Wait. If you have the right talent your turn will come. Imagine you were off on your own—how many fewer cases would you be doing then? How much more overhead would you have to cover all alone? Who would you talk to about difficult cases?"

2. Accept the fact that all partnerships are flawed because all people are flawed. Even the coziest partnerships have a 5 percent grief and regret factor. There's nobody in this business we know who's holding hands with their partners singing hymns around the campfire. Indeed, being an affable partner is something that many eye surgeons have to struggle with for their entire careers, it's their "adapted" personality, not their natural state. The ophthalmic personality is not often given to playing well in groups. On top of all that, ophthalmology is now an increasingly disciplined business. Resources are tapering. Profit margins are shrinking. There are more excuses to pick fights. You need to redouble efforts to admit your own flaws and accept the flaws in your partners.

3. Fighting and conflicts, to a point, are good. But you need to understand and respect your partner's willingness to confront and his natural conflict resolution pace. If you're the kind of person who blows off immediate steam at the first provocation, but settles down quickly, you can get into trouble having a partner who quietly, gradually reaches his boiling point. If your style is to talk everything out in the open, and your partner is more obtuse, you're both going to be frustrated. Discuss your differences and then respect them. This is more easily said than done, obviously. If you're running into chronic strife over differences like these, it may help to have all of the partners (and the administrator and department heads if appropriate) tested with one of the common personality inventories, and then be oriented as a group on the results by a trained professional. It's worth the time commitment—you may just be a few hours away from making your work environment a lot more pleasant.

4. When there's strife, as difficult as it may be, look in the mirror first and ask yourself, "Is it me? Am I causing this?" Ask for and defer to the opinion of a few trusted coaches.

5. Don't use the administrator or other lay staff as the referee for doctor-to-doctor conflict resolution. If you're an office manager and your doctors are in a fight, your first instinct may be to dive in and break up the rumble. You should resist this in most cases. As any police officer can tell you, some of the most dangerous calls they go out on are seemingly minor domestic quarrels. Like an

unwary cop, you can get yourself shot if, as an office manager, you try to resolve partner conflicts that have heated beyond a certain point. Even if you succeed in lowering tensions, at least one of the partners will likely perceive you have taken an opposing side; the resentment will be durable, and you can lose the ability to lead in other areas of the practice in the future. It's far more appropriate for the managing partner or an outside party to rescue difficult situations. Managing partners can be rotated out. An outside consultant can be dismissed and replaced with two phone calls. But losing a valued administrator can set your practice back for years.

6. There's no such thing as a 50-50 partnership. Perfect equality is as much a myth as Santa Claus, another idealistic archetype that serves a valuable social purpose to keep naive believers temporarily in line. Somebody in your practice is the smartest. Somebody is the dumbest. Somebody is the best with financial details. Somebody is the most skilled surgeon. And chances are, nobody is the best at everything. The *TEAM* acronym, "Together Everyone Achieves More," only works if you harness everyone's unique strengths, and simultaneously acknowledge that not everyone is going to get a perfectly fair, perfectly even deal. This year you might earn less, but your partner finally get lanes two and three equipped just the way she wants them. Next year, you can get your LASIK marketing program tuned up, while your partner takes a mild pay cut for you in turn. To be a happy partner, your favorite expression has to become, "I can live with that." Not every partner problem has a solution. Living with a modicum of small inequalities is obligatory.

7. Don't hesitate to call 911. You need to know when partner discord has lasted longer or plunged deeper than is healthy. There are all kinds of outside parties you can draw on, depending on what's at issue. Your accountant might best solve a purely financial argument. Interpersonal frictions and corrosive dishonesties may yield to an industrial psychologist. Practice management consultants typically provide help with multi-disciplinary issues, as when both practice governance and financial integrity have fallen off.

8. Practice divorce is an acceptable, if regrettable and expensive, solution. As we've lectured and written elsewhere, business partnerships are a kind of unconsummated, childless marriage. The relationship glue is your common vision of what you can create together, your stepwise progress, and your fear that practicing outside of partnership will be worse than what you have now. But sometimes even this glue is not strong enough to bond unsuitable partners. If it's at long last time for a practice divorce, make the break as cleanly and as fairly as possible, *but do so only after heroic efforts to work things out, and to understand precisely*

why things failed. Just like the ordinary kind of marriage, your failure to thrive in the current practice marriage will often lead to successive botches.

We hope that with the ideas above, you and your partners will be able to stop well short of divorce. With any luck it may be as easy as ceasing to look so hard for what's wrong, and focus instead on what's right about your partnership. Accentuate the positives. As Ben Franklin might have said, were he an ophthalmologist, "Enter a partnership with crystalline vision and thereafter work hard to develop a progressive case of macular degeneration."

What can be said about partner-partner relationships also applies, in a modified way, of course, to the relationship between employer docs and their junior/employee associates. Why are associates important in the context of a book on cash flow? Because their work provides a source of coverage for fixed overhead, and they can ultimately, be the best source of passive income for practice owners.

Among the many great mysteries of the ophthalmic world, one the most enduring is summarized in the question, "What does my associate doctor want, anyway?" What's left after you feel you've given the moon, the sun and the stars and your employee doctor is still not happy? There's no easy answer, especially when an overly tight senior doctor is the employer of an overly grabby junior doctor. Here's a brief digest of the most common complaints we hear from junior associates, along with a few ideas to help their employers and practice managers.

Broadly, associate doctors, whether permanently slated as associates or on a partner track, want respect. They (at least usually) understand that they are not first in the practice pecking order. But they do want lay support staff to be unresponsive to reasonable requests.

As an owner, foster a group spirit and talk about the "team." Be an "us" practice, not a "me" practice in all communication, at staff meetings, in speaking with patients, and in marketing materials. It's in marketing coverage that some of the rawest conflicts arise, not only interpersonally but also in a very practical business sense. If your practice advertises, we know that using one doctor's name as the name of the practice, like "Michaelson Eye Center," works better than a generic name like "Western Eye Center." And we have also learned that using one doctor spokesperson as the public guarantor of quality works better than a parade of different faces. If your practice can overcome the ego strains, stick to one person in the ads. If the associates insist on their 15 minutes of fame, use a group shot and use the fact that you take a team approach as one factor distinguishing your service.

The highest quality associates want to get involved with decision making and with special projects they can call their own. Allow associates to sit in on non-sensitive portions of your practice's partner meetings. Give them a voice, even if they don't have a vote. There's no need to discard an associate who doesn't volunteer for extra duties like coming eagerly to these meetings. But that behavior may be a signal that the associate is not partner material. By allowing a young doctor to participate in the group's discussions on strategy and spending philosophy today, you help a partner-in-training make better decisions for you in the future.

Doctors who have not yet made partner, along with younger partners, are often exquisitely sensitive about how new patients are assigned in the practice, especially if the compensation methodology leans toward top line production. There should be a written protocol for scheduling new patients, and the front desk or appointment clerks should be checked periodically so that the very human tendency to please the senior partner by feeding her patients does not bias the system.

Most associates, and partners, too, detest clinical pigeonholes and being kept from areas of practice that they enjoy. There are numerous conflicts arising today as the senior doctors in some settings carve out LASIK surgery for themselves (just watch—the tide is turning as procedure fees settle down to earth and it becomes most profitable once again to provide general eye care and cataract surgery!). As a general principle, unless associates are hired with the express agreement that they will stick to defined practice areas, it works best if every doctor is permitted to provide whatever care that they are sufficiently trained to perform.

Even the most junior doctors will commonly—and understandably—complain if they are forced to report solely to a lay manager in the practice, or answer to a clinician or para-professional they deem to be of lower status. We ordinarily construct client organization charts with dual reporting lines so that doctors report to a medical director or managing partner for clinical affairs and to the practice administrator for business matters.

It's not unusual for doctors—even pure, permanent employees—to react adversely when the partner doctors use staff and other practice resources for personal purposes. We're speaking here about the common practice of a senior doctor sending someone out for personal errands or over to their home for childcare or housekeeping duties. It's clearly your right as an owner to deploy staff as you see fit, subject only to your accountant's comfort with this, but try to not rub these perks in your associates' faces. If you are in a closely held practice (where such line blurring between personal and business expenses are most common) be sure to install a charge-back protocol for quasi-business expenses when your associate becomes a partner.

Partner-track associates obviously want an equity stake in the practice. But owners and associates are rarely on the same page regarding a fair percentage. Owners can be too parsimonious, offering just 5 percent or 10 percent, even if their associate does nearly half of the work. We find even more often that it's the associates who are over reaching. It's not unusual during a consulting assignment in this area to speak with an associate who perhaps generates just 20 percent of the practice's revenue but expects to be granted a full 50 percent equity position. If you're an associate surgeon reading this, put yourself in your employer's shoes. The employer is likely either going to want to retain a 51 percent majority control, or at the very least have legal documents obliging a supermajority vote (which is controlled by contract even with a minority position.) Precise fairness to both sides calls for an equity position for all partner providers pro-rata to their revenue or profit contributions, subject only to the preferences of a founding or majority partner, whose word—legally and morally—should be law.

Believe it or not, associate doctors want clear boundaries. A common complaint heard from associates about to be terminated is, "I never knew I was expected to do that. Why didn't somebody tell me?" Every new associate should be given a written summary of your minimum performance expectations. This list may reasonably be quite different for partner-track associates, who should *cheerfully and skillfully* take on extra work in such areas as staff training, community outreach and quality assurance review.

Whether you're an associate or an owner—or a manager stuck in between when these two parties get into conflict—it may help to hand out copies of this chapter to help stimulate a discussion and reach a resolution.

Next to individual doctor productivity, cash flow is most influenced by the work of the practice administrator or office manager. Great lay managers can make mediocre doctors, and their income statements, look great.

Few practices stand still. In the past few years, an increasing number of practices have grown rapidly with continued opportunities for local consolidation. Most practices have at least slowly increased in revenue, size and enterprise complexity. A few spiral downward, either by design (as when a doctor decides to slow down), or by neglect. Whatever the direction of change in your practice, it's statistically unlikely the practice administrator who was a *perfect* fit when they were hired is still well matched today.

The skill set of your practice manager or administrator should be in line with the needs of your practice today, as well as anticipated future needs. Let's say your practice's profit margins have thinned for the past few years. The dip from 50 percent to 40 percent profits might have been barely noticed. But now the margins are approaching just 30 percent, the staff are over-due for another pay raise and your aging office is ready for a facelift. You clearly have a financial problem. And you may need a new administrator or manager, with skill sets that line up with your most pressing kinds of problems. But in this example, you should discriminate. You may need a manager who has sharp accounting skills, who can contain costs. Or, you may really need a manager whose core competency is in marketing, to boost the top line of the practice, which will pump up the bottom line and allow you to afford the new costs.

Here are several warning signs, by no means a complete list, that your ophthalmic practice manager may be in trouble.

1. Your manager lacks a sufficiently broad skill set. No manager is a complete package. The clichés are true: Strength in finance and accounting is classically antithetical to good human resource development skills. A manager with outstanding sales and marketing skills, can be befuddled when looking at the bottom line. And outstanding strategic thinkers often overlook day-to-day operations. But to the extent possible, your manager should have balanced skills, and perhaps more importantly, the ability (and humility) to know when to call on outside expertise.

2. Your manager is not sufficiently committed to his/her career. It's ordinary for a practice manager to spend 50+ hours per week on the job, even in smaller practices. They should be among the first to arrive and among the last to leave. It's rarely helpful for a manager to work part-time and be routinely missing on one or more days per week, unless the rest of the management team (the head tech, optical manager, patient accounts manager, etc.) are extremely high functioning and can work autonomously.

3. Your manager has burned bridges with staff or doctors. Let's face it. Even the smallest practice is an emotionally and politically charged environment. Even superior managers that start out with 100 points may slowly have their leadership capacity diminished by the corrosive barbs of competing staff member or doctors. Enough judgment errors and a harsh physician board may lose sufficient confidence in an administrator to let allow him/her to work independently and do their job.

4. Your manager has simply lost interest. Talented managers need stimulation. If you have a mundane, no-growth practice, your manager may not have enough to do. Finding a special project, or leasing your manager out to referring optometrists as a consultant may perk your manager up. Make sure your practice has objective performance benchmarks, which a manager can strive to reach to relieve their boredom.

5. Your manager is in over his/her head. The signals from a drowning manager are often overlooked. Competence can and should be measured. Are deadlines made, written down and kept? Is your manager in command of the myriad details? Inasmuch as written and verbal skills are at the heart of management, does your manager have the communication skills (including *listening*) to be able to run the practice? Bluntly, are they smart enough for the job?

6. Your manager fails to delegate. Doctors are too quick to applaud super-hero managers who take on every detail of every project. Authority and responsibility should be sufficiently distributed throughout the practice so that no one person is "mission critical."

7. Your manager fails to groom his/her eventual replacement. As vital as an administrator is to your organization, it's critical that this manager work to continuously groom his/her understudy. Mentoring a junior manager in training is understandably skipped by insecure managers and relished by strong, secure managers.

It's quite common for physician-owners to wring their hands and delay making a decision about their faltering manager. Whatever you may say about the perfectionistic tendencies of ophthalmologists, at the core they have soft hearts and an aversion to conflict, which can drag out the "What are we going to do with Francis?!?" decision. When doing administrative remediation and recruitment work for clients, one of the first questions we explore is "How long has your current manager's performance been unsatisfactory?" The answer commonly exceeds a year.

The strongest practices don't make any fewer senior management hiring blunders, but they do make their mistakes faster and are willing to fix or cut an under-performing manager. It may be perceived kindness to give "Francis" yet another try, but at the same time you may have 10, 20 or more staff members and their families (not to mention your own!) dependent on optimal performance at the top. It's lax leadership to put 10 or 20 careers in jeopardy just to avoid one confrontation. And such confrontation needn't lead to termination.

It may be that your now under-performing manager was elevated to his/her position just a little too soon. Find an honorable way for them to step back into a more junior role for a few quarters or years. If your practice has grown rapidly, outpacing the career development pace of your relatively junior office manager, the easiest solution may be to bring in a more seasoned administrator, and let that individual determine the best slot for your out-paced manager.

Perhaps your manager does not perform satisfactorily simply because he/she doesn't have performance guidelines. The basics should include a position description, a written set of operational enhancement goals for the next year, and specific financial targets for the practice. If your administrator doesn't have a roadmap and directions from the doctors, he/she is likely to drive your practice to an unintended financial or strategic destination.

Practices are more complex, and have more moving parts, today than ever before. Happily, most managers, with the help of groups like the American Society of Ophthalmic Administrators and the Medical Group Management Association, have all the resources they need to stay ahead.

The most common skill deficit we see for working managers (most of whom have come up through the ranks of the practice, and not through formal business training) is in the area of finance, accounting, and budgeting. As fees slip and profit margins thin, it's imperative that both managers and managing partners develop real skills in this area.

When it's time for a new manager, the typical, small (2-5 doctor) group practice is exchanging a $45,000-55,000 per year office manager for a $75,000-plus per year administrator. This fact should feel as threatening to the under-performing manager as it feels encouraging to strong managers. For practices, there is an increasing mandate to secure competent management staff, because practices within competitive markets are no longer just competing doctor-to-doctor, but manager-to-manager for dominance.

Managers must be given the time and dollar resources to attend meetings, take field trips to other successful practices, and purchase study materials. This, combined with higher base salaries, and an increasing trend toward bonus compensation—and even equity participation by superior managers—is driving up costs for practices. Often as not, this cost has a great, ultimate financial return. We believe this will continue to contribute to a trend of the aggregation of some smaller practices into larger practices—organizations that can collectively afford exceptional management talent.

Increasingly, the practice with an under-performing manager will simply lack the one strategic asset that is increasingly the most needed to stay ahead, even if this same practice has superior clinicians, superior equipment, a great team of support staff and a long history of past successes.

Most eye surgeons, partnered or solo, live in an eat-what-you-kill world. Virtually all of their income is *active*, that is, they only gain in profitability if they work harder and are capped by the number of hours in a day. How can entrepreneurial eye doctors best harness the *passive* income opportunities used in every other business sector?

Surgery centers and optical dispensing are a start, but as revenue per RVU stagnates over the years ahead and costs inexorably rise, the only surgeons with a shot at historic income levels will be those who develop strong local brands, gain control over patient distribution channels (read: managed care contracting, consumer advertising or optometric referral control), and employ other doctors to provide a passive income stream.

Ultimately, like so much of your professional life, it all comes down to discipline. You need to have the discipline to examine thoroughly where you really stand and where the trends are taking you. You need to have the foresight to not be an ostrich and assume you'll somehow muddle through as you always have in the past. The last decade of Medicare fee reductions have been nibbles compared to the considerable "chomps" ahead of us. You need to have the discipline to admit to your soft points, and commit to their improvement.

With any luck, by taking lots of small incremental steps, year by year, you'll stay ahead of the falling fee curve…and you'll stay ahead of the doctors to the left and right of you in town. You had better assume that they are reading this book and tuning up their games, too.

Chapter Nine:
Cash Flow Smoke Alarms—Graphical Analysis and Benchmarking

As an administrator or practice owner, do you sometimes feel you get the run-around from your patient accounts management staff? Or perhaps you're an associate surgeon in a practice and you're paid based on a percentage of your collections. How confident are you that staff does everything possible to collect for all the hard work you've done? As the manager of the billing department, do you find it hard to communicate with your administrator or doctors about the status of your department's progress? Well, this chapter is for all of you.

Too often, when doctors and managers gather and discuss the state of the billing department, the conversation goes like this:

Dr. Witherholt: "So how are we doing on collections, Susan?"

Susan: "Just great doctor! My staff are working hard, and I've cancelled vacations until we can bring the receivables down just a little bit. The new computer system is still a pain, but the vendor is finally returning my calls. And did you hear that TrueCare is finally paying us after all those re-submissions? Thanks, by the way, for getting better at signing off your superbills."

What's missing in all this happy chatter? The *numbers*! As the saying goes, talk is cheap because the supply exceeds the demand. If Susan's description of her department's progress moves beyond the subjective to the numeric facts, two important things start to happen. First, Susan becomes more accountable for the performance of her team. It's all too easy even for competent managers to develop poor habits if they are not challenged by the owners to delivery the details. It may be uncomfortable the first few times to confess to any negative collection trends. But exposing the problems precisely—and that means numerically—is the start of marshalling the resources you need for a solution. Second, the managing doctor rapidly becomes a better owner of the practice, more willing to loosen the purse strings when billing managers ask for more staff time, training and computer power. With reliable numbers, owners know the results of these expensive, additional resources are going to be *measurable*.

Now imagine a different doctor-manager conversation:

Dr. Witherholt: So how are we doing on collections, Susan?

Susan: "Just great doctor! It's all in my report to the board, but I can tell you that in the last six months our accounts receivable ratio (the month-ending total A/R divided by average monthly charges) has fallen from 2.3 to 1.7. Our over-90-day receivables have dropped below 20 percent of our total A/R, which was the maximum threshold we set as a department policy. You'll recall that we had a resubmission rate of 18 percent. That has now dropped to about 5 percent in a typical month because the front desk crew is better at entering the patient demographics right the first time. Although we haven't changed our charge levels or service mix, our collection ratio has climbed in the last year from 56 percent to 67 percent. Now that we've worked through the old receivables backlog, the labor costs in my department are coming down. We're now collecting an annualized $1.1 million per full-time-equivalent staff member on our team—that's up 25 percent from when I took over the department."

Wow! Some difference, huh? Which of these two, very different conversations go on in your practice today? From these two extremely contrasting examples, you can begin to see how important the numbers are.

And what really helps is to put these numeric trends in their historic trend context with simple graphs. Here are a few examples from an imaginary practice that needs a little work:

This A/R aging graph shows you the status of each aging bucket. As you can see, the 120+ day receivables have started to come down, but the 90+ day figure is growing. This commonly happens when patient accounts staff focus on one problem, while they let other areas slip.

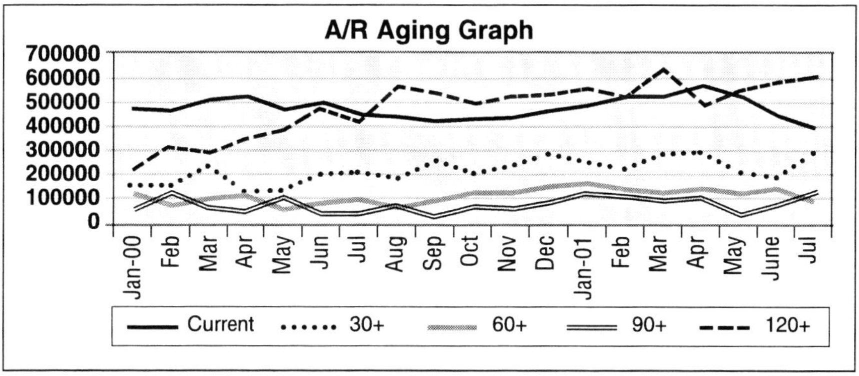

As you can see from this graph, the percent of receivables over 90 days is coming down, but still significantly exceed normal limits. Agreed thresholds, along with longer-term graphs like this, shared with the patient accounts staff each month, can help motivate and track progress.

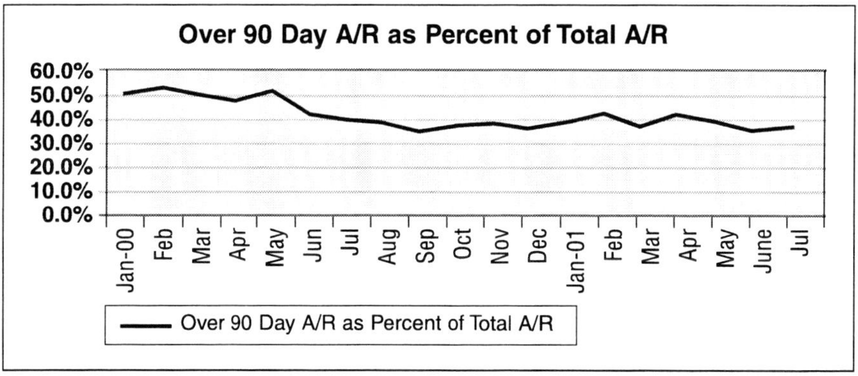

Your practice can set agreed standards for where receivables should float in relationship to average monthly charges, and then compare this ideal figure graphically to the actual A/R. For a Medicare-dominated general ophthalmology practice, having 1.8-times average monthly charges or less reflected as a total A/R figures is a reasonable benchmark. As this sample graph shows, our imaginary practice has recently improved. Reviewing this graph each month would provide an early warning system if receivables ever fell out of line again.

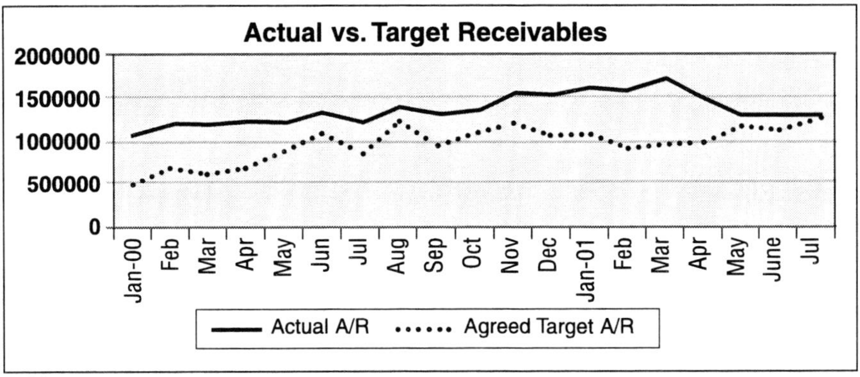

Here's another way to express with a simple graph the degree to which the practice's A/R is out of bounds. This graph can be very motivating to billing staff.

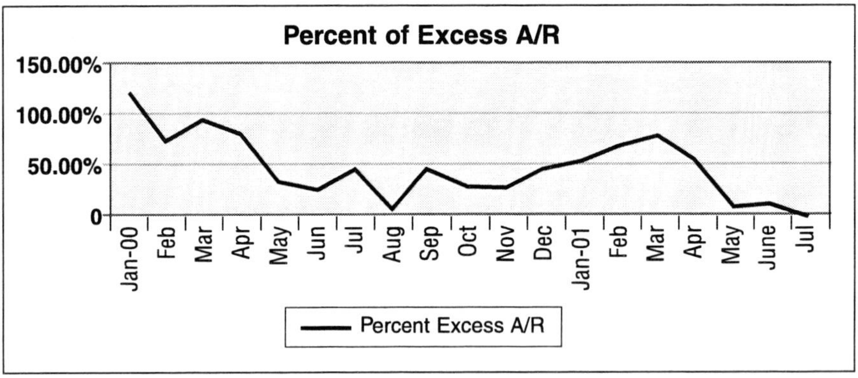

Keep in mind that all of these numeric examinations can be performed not only on the practice-at-large, but also on individual segments. You can examine and graph the relevant figures for an individual distant satellite office to see if the decentralized billing staff in this location have met standards set by the home office. If you're an associate paid a percentage of your collections, you can drill down into the data to see if your individual accounts are being worked hard or hardly worked.

The term, "the whole nine yards" came from World War II fighter pilots doing battle in the Pacific theater. When arming their airplanes on the ground, the .50 caliber machine gun ammunition belts measured exactly 27 feet before being loaded into the fuselage. If the pilots fired all of their ammo at a target, it got, "the whole nine yards."

Clearly, very few practices go "the whole nine yards" when trying to get paid for the work their doctors do. One part of finding out just where you stand in the complex collections process is to measure the collection ratio—that portion of gross charges that you have received. It's the simple decimal or percentile figure that results by dividing collections by charges. This ratio can be gathered over the course of a month, a quarter or even a year. But it's far more valuable when looked at month-by-month over longer time periods…18 to 24 months is about right.

Let's examine this important cash flow index, the collection ratio, in your practice, and what it can tell you about the efficiency of you and your billing staff. It's important to point out that the actual decimal or percentile number can be quite different from practice to practice. In a practice with extremely high charges (and correspondingly high write-offs) the collection ratio may be low. In practices with charges that are closer to allowable fees, the collection ratio is higher. High or low, what we're looking for here is not the number, but the trend in the number. Once collections are handled correctly, you then want to see stability in the collection ratio, unless, of course you change your fees or payers' allowables change. When you graph monthly collections divided by charges, what you see may look something like this:

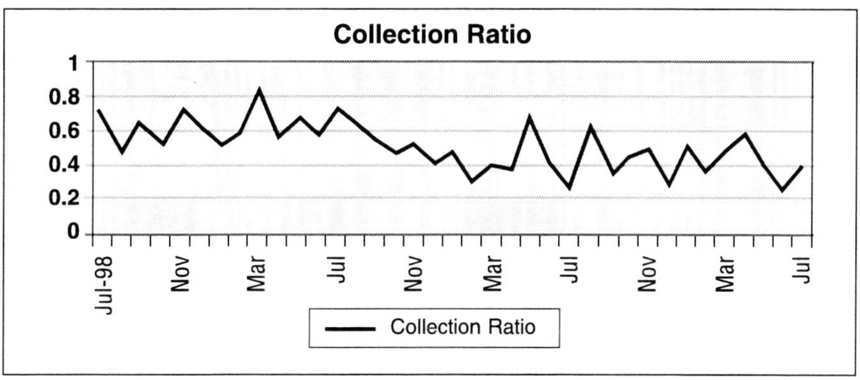

Obviously, in this graph, the trend line is adverse—the collection ratio has become smaller. The doctors are paid a smaller and smaller percent of every dollar they submit as a claim. This is not the graph you want to see in your practice.

Here's another graph, from an entirely different client setting. In this practice, efforts were taken at several levels to make sure that collections were maximized.

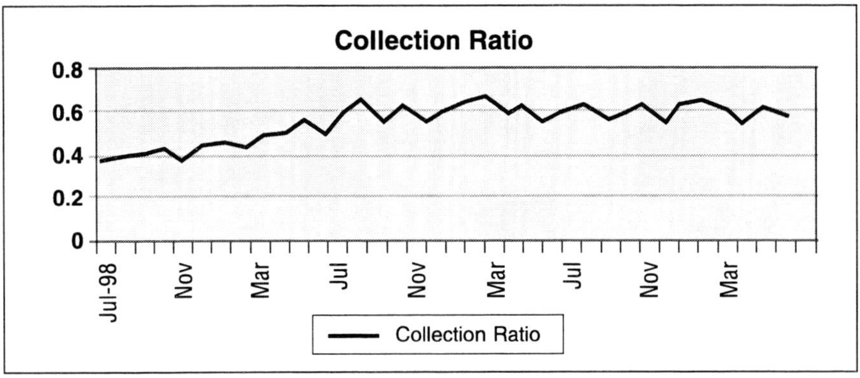

These trends, down in the first collection ratio graph and up in the second, can be due to a number of factors. In recent years, the most common increase in a practice's collection ratio has been related to the addition of LASIK, elective plastics, or optical dispensing. Because each of these services are typically reimbursed at or near 100 percent of charges, the collection ratio can skew upward. It may be appropriate in mixed practice settings to break out the graphs so you can see each disparate segment on its own.

Another change that elevates collection ratios has been hitting practices with modest surgical volumes for the past several years as allowable fees have slowly crept up for cognitive services, and slipped lower (or at least not risen as fast) for most procedures. So if yours is a younger practice, seeing more and more surgical volume every year, your collection ratio may actually be slipping. Not to worry. At the other end of the career spectrum, don't be surprised if, as you perform less and less surgery, your personal collection ratio increases slightly.

An improving collection ratio can be due to little more than a change in payer mix. If you've been largely a Medicare provider in the past and have finally been admitted as a provider for a popular private insurance plan paying more than Medicare allowable rates, your collection ratio will increase if you have just one fee schedule.

Changes in surgical density can change your collection ratio. For example, even if you are not shifting from cataract surgery to LASIK or the reverse, a shift to higher case volumes (especially if you maintain extremely high charges for cataract sur gery to take advantage of one or two high-paying private insurance payers), may actually decrease your collection ratio.

Collection ratios can also slip slightly when the check out staff become less aggressive in asking for patient-responsible amounts. It's reasonable to verify daily that the front desk has stayed on top of requests and receipts of co-payments, deductibles and refraction fees. A simple daily log of window payments, or window payments divided by patient visits (if your patient volume fluctuates) can help to flag when this dimension of collections is faltering. Of course, you can take auditing in this area to its extreme limit and check what percent of the actual expected amount you collected.

A negligent billing department is the most common reason for collections to drop; the collection ratio graph is an outstanding monitor for performance of this part of the practice team. When a patient accounts/billing department is overwhelmed, not only does the collection ratio drop, but the older collections work goes undone. When you first suspect the billing department has fallen behind, immediately check the A/R ratio (month-ending A/R divided by the average of the last three month's charges). It should be under 2.0 for a general ophthalmology practice, and under 1.5 for a mixed LASIK/cataract practice. Then check the aged trial balance report. The over-90-day amounts should not exceed 18-20 percent of the total A/R in a general practice.

What goal should you set for your collection ratio? For the typical general ophthalmology practice, 55 percent-65 percent is the norm. Again, any time you change fees, up or down, there will be change in your collection ratio. An increase in gross fees charged will decrease the collection ratio, and vice-versa. Some volatility is also introduced by the fact that you generally collect in month two and three for work performed in month one. An alternative to graphing collections divided by gross charges is to graph collections divided by *allowable* charges. This is called the net collection ratio. In this case, the ratio should reach 1.0 (100 percent in percentile terms). However, as with all practice ratios, it's best to compare yourself internally over time rather than benchmarking to some national average.

If you are just one surgeon in a large multi-subspecialty (eye only) or multi-specialty practice, and you suspect that your collections are low, it can be useful to look at your individual collection ratio, compared to your ophthalmic peers. Several times a year we consult with surgeons that are part of a large clinic department and concerned that their institution's billing department does not do their part to handle collections. Half of the time they're right; the rest of the time, it's actually errors, omissions, and delays from individual doctors that are holding up collections.

The value of graphing various performance benchmarks in your practice over time using Microsoft Excel or a similar spread sheeting/graphing program hugely exceeds the time it takes to learn how to use these programs and enter the data each month. Yet it's only a minority of practices that take the trouble to do so. Think of these graphs as a kind of "smoke alarm" for the practice. Just like the alarm in your house, when the alarm goes off you know that something is amiss and you set out a room-to-room search. Precisely the same department-to-department search needs to occur when your practice's patient accounts' alarm goes off. In the next chapter, we'll cover a very logical, step-by-step approach to tracking down the source of the problems that often first become visible when you generate these performance graphs.

If you're ready for the advanced version of this chapter, consider additional graphing and other checks:

- Prepare a two-line graph showing over the past 18-24 months two data points for each month: The profit available for shareholder doctor distribution; and the actual amount of such distributions. For a practice with poor discipline, salaries and other officer entitlements can outstrip available cash, and the owners are left to live on their bank lines and their vendor's stretched out credit terms.

- Divide the monthly cost to run the core practice (not including optical or ASC segments, and not including doctor distributions and depreciation) by the monthly patient counts, and prepare a multi-year graph showing the trend on this number. There is a wide range between practices, from about $50 to well over $100.

- Graph lay support staff costs per patient visit over many months to check for trends in labor productivity. Increasing productivity can potentially substantiate pay raises. Falling rates may suggest cuts. Beware, in large, old, generous, and permissive practices you'll find mounting labor costs that attend such inattention and largesse. The legacy costs of high-tenure staff, hired in the fat years of the profession, can (and will increasingly in the future) usher practices into bankruptcy.

- Track visual fields, angiography and other special testing as a percent of total patient visits to track trends in utilization. Both over and under utilization are cause for concern.

- Track optical sales as a percent of total practice sales or optical sales per average patient visit.

- Divide the number of billing department payroll hours each month by the number of patient visits in the same month. We've seen practices pay as much as 1.5 staff payroll hours per patient visit, which is a sure sign of inefficiency. Norms are 0.3 or lower.

- Look each month at trends in total collections per billing department full-time equivalent.

- Graph adjustments each month. Volatility in this figure may point out periods of inattention followed by periods of excessive write-offs to catch up. The curve should be fairly stable in an otherwise stable practice.

- Prepare a weekly or monthly claims denial report showing by doctor the number and dollar amounts and reasons for each denied claim; this can help point out individual doctor mistakes that are slowing cash flow:

Month of:	**Doctor Smith**		**Doctor Jones**	
Reason For Denial	Number of Denials	Dollar Amount Denied	Number of Denials	Dollar Amount Denied
Not received by payer				
Wrong payer				
Policy number in error				
No authorization				
Coding error				
Misc Clinic Errors				
Misc Payer Errors				
Total				

Most patients' accounts teams actually do an outstanding, even heroic job for their practices but are under-appreciated. So one of the side benefits of a little extra graphing work each month, even if all the numbers are positive, is to get the respect and recognition you deserve. If you're an administrator or manage the receivables for your practice, commit today to holding yourself and your team accountable to these higher standards of review. If you're a practice owner, insist on these standards. And then be *sure* to reward your people when they deliver the numbers.

Chapter Ten: Patient Accounts Engineering— Developing Process Standards and Scorecards

As if ophthalmic medicine and surgery were not already maddeningly precise and complex, the business side of ophthalmology contains thousands of small moving parts, too. Many of these small parts are in turn only driven by a well-oiled composite of trained staff resources, emerging computer technology, and regulatory oversight. In this chapter we present a few evaluation and management tools for your patient accounts department.

It's a wonder that most practices manage to get most of the operational wrinkles ironed out, at least most of the time. The most frequent—and most expensive—wrinkles that remain are in the day-to-day management of the practice's patient accounts.

We all like filling out those simple magazine quizzes, you know, the ones that tell us where we stand on our fitness, our intelligence, or our love life. Here's the same kind of quick quiz that you can apply to your reception and patient accounts department. While the scorecard below obviously does not point out every missing nuance, it's a very useful one-time or ongoing gross measure of the kind of job this department is doing. And it can get people in your practice talking about where efforts to improve cash flow should first be applied.

PATIENT ACCOUNTS MANAGEMENT SCORECARD

Patient Accounts Area	Scoring (points 1-6)	Practice Score
Distribution of patient accounts and computer skills in the practice	1=only one or two insurance clerks know how to post charges and submit and follow up claims 3=in addition, office manager knows how to enter charges, submit claims and run reports 6=in addition, doctors know how to enter charges, submit claims and run reports	
Billing Staff Ratio—I (annual total practice collections divided by the number of billing staff full-time equivalents)	1=under $800,000 3=$800,000 - $1.2 million 5=over $1.2 million (Note: this metric is highly variable depending on the average charge and managed care demands of the market…a Lasik or retinal practice may be normal at over $1.5 million in collections per FTE-year)	
Billing Staffing Ratio—II (patient accounts staff annual payroll hours, divided by the number of annual total patient visits plus surgical cases)	1=over 0.30 payroll hours per [visits+cases] 2=0.30 payroll hours per [visits+cases] 3=under 0.30 payroll hours per [visits+cases] (Note: this metric is highly variable depending on the experience, work intensity and managed care demands of the market)	
Patient accounts computer system	1=current computer is outdated or outgrown, or is a new platform with few users 3=current computer is off-brand, but works well enough 5=current computer, whether in-house or through a billing service, is among the top systems used nationally and it works well	
Coding/Charting/Billing consultation	1=no external consulting review 2=periodic external review (every 4+ yrs) 3=external review at least every 2-3 yrs	
Compliance program	1=there is no formal or informal compliance program in place 2=a somewhat informal compliance program is in place but we are less serious about this than we should be 3=a formal compliance program is in place with an appropriate depth of oversight	
Coordination between billing and reception staff	1=poor coordination 3=fair coordination 5=good or better coordination	
Patient demographics entered accurately and completely	1=over 25 percent inaccuracies or refiled claims 3= 6-24 percent inaccuracies or refiled claims 5=under 5 percent inaccuracies or refiled claims	
Missing ticket reports	1=no check for missing tickets 2=periodic check for missing tickets 3=daily missing ticket report	

Superbill filled out accurately and completely, preferably by doctor	1=the superbill has to be returned to doctors or staff for completion or clarification several times a day 3=several times a week superbills have to be taken back to doctors or staff 5=with very few exceptions, the superbill is complete and accurate	
Coding levels	1=the practice routinely over-codes and is currently at risk for an adverse audit 3=the practice routinely under-codes to "play it safe" 5=with rare exceptions, the practice codes at a level appropriate to the diagnosis and services rendered	
Charges posted accurately, preferably by front desk at checkout	1=it commonly takes over 24 hours from the time of service to post a charge in our computer 2=charges are nearly always posted within 24 hours of service 3=charges are always posted on the same day	
Fee schedules	1=many of our fees are below those allowed by our payer contracts; we never compare payments allowed to our contracts, and have not reviewed our fee schedule for more than a year 3=most of our fees are appropriate, but there are isolated instances of our fees being below the amount allowed by payers; we should probably revise our fee structure 5=our gross fees are reviewed at least annually, and are uniformly above those allowed by third-party payers	
Window payments	1=the practice receives under 50 percent of what it should collect from patients at the time of service (co-pays, deductibles, refraction fees, glasses deposits, etc.) Staff must often bill for these small amounts. 2=the practice only collects about 50 percent to 90 percent of what it should at the time of service 3=the practice receives more than 90 percent of patient-responsible amounts at the time of service; we may have to be a little more diligent with patient refunds for over-payments, but we only rarely have to bill patients	
Timely claims submission	1=all claims are routinely submitted more than 72 hours after services are rendered; some claims are delayed much longer 2=most claims go out 24 to 72 hours after services are rendered 3=virtually all electronic claims are submitted daily and within 24 hours of services rendered; paper claims are submitted at least twice a week	

Electronic claims submission	1=all claims are paper, even though some electronic claims are possible 2=not all possible opportunities for electronic claims are taken 3=all possible claims are submitted electronically	
Direct deposit of payments	1=although direct deposit is possible, we receive checks 2=we don't use direct deposit options as much as we could 3=all possible payments are received by direct deposit into our bank account	
Timely payment processing	1=payments are posted and secondary claims are submitted only after 48-72 hours or more have passed 2= payments are posted and secondary claims are submitted within 24-48 hours of a check/EOB arriving 3= payments are posted and secondary claims are submitted within 0-24 hours of a check/EOB arriving	
Timely deposit of payments	1=Deposits are made fewer than 3 times a week, and checks sometimes gather up for several days or more 2=Deposits are made 3-4 times a week, and within 48 hours of receipt of funds 3=Deposits are made daily and within 24 hours of receipt of funds	
Collection ratio (monthly collections divided by monthly gross charges)	1=the collection ratio varies wildly from month-to-month, due to swings in work efficiency eg: 30 percent in some months, 90 percent in others. Staff end up getting well under 90 percent of the allowable charges 2=the collection ratio varies somewhat from month to month; we likely get 90-95 percent of the total allowable charges 3=the collection ratio is stable from month to month, and within norms based on the relationship between the fees charged, the allowable charges, and the practice's service mix, typically 50-75 percent, and practice ends up getting at least 95 percent of the total allowable charges	
A/R Ratio (Total receivables divided by avg of last 3 months)	1=over 2.1 2=1.8-2.0 3=under 1.8 (note: this ratio is applicable to practices with a single, high fee schedule that approximates payments made by the most generous private carriers. This ratio is much lower in practices with two fee schedules, one for Medicare, and a second, higher schedule for non-Medicare)	

Aged trial balance report	1=never produced or reviewed 2=produced and reviewed periodically 3-produced monthly and reviewed by doctors, administrator and billing staff	
Billing department division of labor	1=work is concentrated so that the loss of one staff member leaves a large gap (eg: one staff in charge of all Medicare claims) 2=mild degree of cross-training; the practice is somewhat vulnerable to the loss of a single key staff member 3=avid cross-training; ideally, in larger practices, patient accounts work is divided alphabetically by patient name so that all staff are interchangeable	
Billing integrity audits	1=patient charts, super-bills and posted charges are never cross-checked 3=clinical, front desk and patient accounts team work is rarely checked to make sure all the myriad steps are followed to secure payment for practice services 5= patient charts, super-bills and posted charges are cross-checked daily; laser and special testing equipment logs are compared to charges posted weekly; submission audits are done to make sure submissions are timely and all according to a written protocol	
Progressive internal collection efforts with patients	1=the same statements are sent over and over with no sense of progressive urgency 2=when our older patient-responsible accounts seriously back up and as time permits, the practice works to follow up with these delinquent patients 3=letters, stickers or statement notes, along with follow up calls, are used to incrementally warn delinquent patients	
Collection agencies	1=the practice has no internal or external collection agency; once patients decline payment, the matter is dropped 2=the practice has a collection agency, but it is little used because the doctors don't want to annoy patients 3=the practice sends all appropriate patients to an effective collection agency after the doctor has signed off the chart	
"Warning Systems" in place to catch problems early	1=Billing trends (collection ratio, A/R ratio, days in A/R, billing staff productivity, etc.—see Chapter Nine) are never examined, either internally, or against national benchmarks 2= Billing trends are seldom compared, internally, or against national benchmarks; we catch problems months after they arise	

	3=Billing trends are graphed monthly and compared to internal and national benchmarks...we know immediately if we're getting into trouble and why	
	Total Score (maximum possible = 100)	

90 to 100: Excellent work; simply focus on polishing any areas that fall below the top score.
80 to 89: Good work; prepare a plan to improve to the next level.
70 to 79: Average work; practice cash flow is likely to be well under its potential.
Under 70: Poor work; remedial efforts are needed immediately.

Now let's get a little more elaborate. Below is a sample Patient Accounts Flowsheet that can be generated on Word for Windows™ (or any off-the-shelf word processing software) as a tool to help blueprint a practice's patient accounting diligence, and to help staff develop and maintain their own internal standards.

Notice in this that we cover many of the same areas as in the quiz above. But rather than a simple raw score, you have a chance here to measure your performance against standards that you set on your own, for your own unique practice demands. Used effectively, this tool can then help you create an improvement program, with a high degree of accountability for each responsible staff member. Feel free to add or subtract areas in the left hand column to review and improve with this tool.

On the next page is an example abstracted from a typical client setting.

PATIENT ACCOUNTS FLOWSHEET

Area	Current Status	Reasonable Standard	Resources needed	Deadline	Person Responsible
Accurate patient data entered at reception	We are about 70 percent correct (we know this because we have 160 re-filed claims per month)	90 percent	Study the source of errors, set standards and train to these standards; maintain ongoing daily checks. Merge the reception and patient accounts departments, which are now separate	100 days	Mary now; a joint department head in the future
Pre-certification and authorization	Denials are scant; work done 2-14 days in advance	Same	Cross-train to prevent future key staff dependency; get better communication from doctors to staff while the patient is still in the office	Ongoing	Susan
Patients educated regarding their benefits and responsibility to pay	Patients are "clueless"	Patients are knowledge-able	Educational flyers, both a generic piece and one for each major payer	60 days	Bill
Reporting line authority clarity e.g. Do we know who reports to whom?	Moderately misunderstood reporting lines continue, especially between Mary and Susan	All staff clear about reporting lines	Organization chart posted and memo sent to clarify roles, position descriptions for all, question and answer guide covering the most common examples	60 days	Mary
Utilization and practice patterns set by providers and checked against actual practice	There are no written protocols; good consistency by Dr. Wilson, who is solo, but potential for difficulty with the new associate	One agreed best way to do everything in the practice.	Written testing and treatment protocols for the most common presenting conditions and Return to Clinic standards set and kept; performance checked periodically against these standards.	180 days	Dr. Wilson
Coding/charting consistency and correctness	There are no written standards and many missed charges.	Coding and charting standards are kept high and known to all staff.	Written standards developed; train to these standards; daily routine chart reviews by a designated internal auditor.	90 days	Mary
Patient responsible amounts collected at time of service	80 percent or less	90 percent or higher	Study each office to measure the actual potential recovery rates vs. current amounts, set standards and awareness for staff, prepare checkout scripts, make sure patients are aware of their financial responsibilities at check-in (or before); periodic spot checks.	45 days	Each satellite facility site manager

Charges posted. Are they timely and accurate?	Clinic charges are now batched and posted within 48 hours; surgical charges are posted within 5 days.	Post each patient's charges at the time of checkout Post surgical charges within 24 hours	Faster doctor surgical dictation, establish written standards and train to these, increase accuracy by having the patient accounts team adjacent to the chart room so that charts are handy for reference; periodic audits and inspections to assure accurate posting.	60 days	Susan
Charges checked vs. laser logs?	No checks, because there is no log on the lasers.	Logs on every unit and a weekly cross-check against charges.	Install logs, and send copy of logs to billing, or send copy of billing to Dave for check against his logs?	10 days	Dave
Claims submitted	Daily	Daily	Sustain excellent work!	Ongoing	Karen
Payments posted and deposited.	Daily	Daily	Check: Will our commercial bank supply a courtesy courier for daily pickup? Can we get an automatic deposit service from our larger payers?	Ongoing	Susan
Secondaries filed	Within 48 hours	Same-day	Check on computer upgrades to simplify submissions.	30 days	Susan
Denials formally reviewed, and resubmitted, appealed or written off.	Denials examined periodically when the doctors ask about them.	Monthly formal review of denials; reasons for denials tabulated each month by doctor and internal problems solved.	Establish a regular monthly meeting, out of which is issued a regular report to the doctors. Whenever we get behind in this area, devote needed staff resources to catch up with the backlog. (Getting behind on this can be a core contributor to the run-up in 90+day accounts)	Ongoing	Karen
Periodic or all-chart reviews	20 charts reviewed every 2 months	Daily review of all charts, appointment schedules and superbills.	Trial audit to identify actual error rate; consider full-time inspector if significant problems.	90 days	Susan
Managed care contract review process.	No review to assure that amounts contracted for are actually paid.	Contracts reviewed and compared to amounts paid.	Review of all contracts now, and ongoing check of payments made	30 days	Dave

Managed care contract officer	None	One person who stays in contact with all payers and seeks new contracts and better terms.	New part-time coordinator, a former assistant hospital administrator, will be hired on a consulting basis.	90 days	Susan
Older accounts status	48 percent of total receivables are in the 90+ day column	At or under 18 percent past 90 days	Since the current patient accounts team of three people is on top of current work but unable to get through the backlog (which has existed chronically for more than two years), hire 1.5 FTEs to clean out the backlog within 6 months. Then, shift these workers to other areas of the practice.	180 days	Susan

Transcribe the basic contents of this table to your own word processor, and fill in the blanks after your practice's benchmarks in each area are determined and reasonable performance standards and deadlines are established to reach them.

By getting a handle on current performance, making your practice's new patient accounts operating standards known and transparent to all doctors and staff, and then living up to them, you'll accelerate cash flow and eliminate the unpleasant experience of feeling chronically behind in this deeply complex area of the practice.

Finally, here is a basic service vs. charge integrity audit tool you can customize to your practice's needs and use to find out just how much you're losing through loose operating standards.

Practice Service vs. Charge Integrity Audit

Instructions: Make 20 copies of this master form for each provider in the practice. This sample size may be expanded if desired. Pull 20 random charts of patients who were most recently seen in the clinic between one and three months ago. This time frame is chosen because all charging activity issued from this visit is likely to be completed, and yet the visit is still recent enough to reflect the current pattern of operations in the billing office and clinic.

Two staff members working side-by-side, one of whom should be a qualified coder, and one an experienced tech or scribe (or doctor) should be selected to review each chart, each corresponding superbill, and each patient accounts computer record. Fill in the relevant information below for each visit. Add all the missed or excess collections, and divide by the number of charts reviewed to get the average missing/excess collections per chart.

Multiply this average missing/excess collections per chart by the total patient visits per year to get the annual impact of errors in the practice. Use this figure for coaching doctors and staff toward tighter performance, keeping in mind that no practice achieves 100 percent accuracy. Repeat periodically, with a greater or larger sample size, as appropriate. The most common errors are doctors forgetting to check off the superbill for all services, and staff making charge entry errors.

Doctor Name:____________________________ Location: ________________

Date of Audit________________

Patient Account Number _____________________ Patient Age____________

Third Party Payer____

Date of Office Visit ___________ Chief Complaint_____________________

Primary Diagnosis____

Secondary Diagnosis____

Services Provided According to What's Documented in the Chart

____

Services Provided According to What's on the Superbill

____

Services Provided According to What's in the Computer

____

(What we actually charged out to the patient or third-party payer)

Charge Error Summary	Estimated Excess Dollars Collected For This Patient Visit	Estimated Under-collection of Dollars For This Patient Visit
Missing codes for services we rendered but did not charge		
Downcoding Errors (resulting in insufficient charges to patients and payers)		
Service codes charged out without substantiation (resulting in excess charges to patients and payers)		
Upcoding Errors (resulting in excess charges to patients and payers)		
Total Dollar Impact		

Chapter Eleven:
Marketing—The Longest Crank on The Great Cash Flow Machine

A consultant and friend named Ed Doyle, who helped found and advise several high tech health companies, always used to say, "Marketing is the crank on your company's cash flow machine." And it's true. Looked at less colorfully, but helpfully, because it begins to define tactics that work as opposed to fluff that doesn't, is that marketing is "*establishing and maintaining an exchange relationship.*"

We talked in Chapter One about the importance of getting relationships, and then pushing as much as ethically possible down that relationship pipeline. In this chapter, we'll talk about what works and what doesn't work in marketing, the latter is especially important in cash flow terms, because practices don't have marketing money to burn as they did in years past.

Many practices today are now headed by younger surgeons (and their young administrators) who were not around in 1977, when it finally became legal for doctors to promote themselves through advertising. Until 1977, laws stood on the books that prohibited professionals of every stripe from describing their services to the public. The original Supreme Court case that allowed lawyers to advertise, as a matter of First Amendment rights to free speech, opened the door to both doctors and hospitals.

Back then, ophthalmology practices ran 70 percent profit margins by providing $2,000 cataract surgery. There was plenty of money left on the table to experiment with marketing, and plenty of room for error. There's little room for error today. Media costs have shot up, at the same time that fees and profits have fallen. Many practices in the late 80's and throughout the 90's, that tried to sustain large volumes based on advertising alone, without a simultaneous improvement in customer service, have had to revise their service model or go out of business. Getting a new patient to enter your practice through paid advertising is more difficult and expensive than ever before, which is why greater attention must now be given to alumni referral development, contract development, patient satisfaction and cross-selling ancillary services to the patients you already have. Not to say that there isn't a large role that paid marketing can play, when clustered with other tactics.

After helping clients spend over $100 million on eye care marketing in the past 25 years, we've had some very expensive lessons about what works and what doesn't. By applying this experience to your own practice, you can shave costs and shorten your own learning curve. Both are vital for survival in today's unforgiving environment, where few practices have the time or capital for mistakes.

Marketing is often pigeon holed as "advertising," "selling," or any of the hundreds of other individual marketing tools. Instead, think of marketing as an entire toolbox. Like a skilled mechanic, the smartest practices take out just the right combination of tools for the job—not too few, not too many, and use them with just the right force—to efficiently establish new patient relationships and to maintain relationships with established patients. These new and ongoing exchange relationships are the soul of all great ophthalmic marketing, no matter what tools are used. Too often the most aggressive practices forget the "maintaining" part of marketing. Nothing makes a poor product fail faster than great advertising—the kind of advertising that gets you loads of new patients, which you then service poorly. Finding a new patient to enter your practice will always be far more expensive than retaining the patients you already have. <u>Retaining</u> happy patients will always be at the core of medical marketing.

Marketing research is critical. You need to <u>think</u> about your audience and marketing before you engage any tactics. Of course, many practices take it in reverse, cranking out half-baked marketing executions, and then scratching heads to figure out why it didn't work.

If your practice had Coca Cola's research budget, you would have a blue print of the motivations and hot buttons of each segment of your patient base. While you'll never have the luxury of this kind of insight, much of what works in ophthalmic marketing can be discovered with simpler and less costly research endeavors, and by applying your experience and common sense. After all, as a surgeon you have intimate contact with each one of your customers—not so the corporate brand manager who has to derive second-hand customer data to understand who's buying his product.

Start by doing a better job inquiring how new patients heard about your practice and the multiple sources influencing their decision to seek treatment. Even in practices where the front desk staff ask the right questions during registration, and actually enter the data in the appropriate field, the resulting monthly management reports are often expressed in terms of charges for just that month by the referral source of all patients, both new and returning. This generally provides misleading, often understated, information about the return on your marketing investments or the life-time cash that flows from a new patient who joins the practice.

Instead, the data you need most emerges from this question: "What's the *anticipated total future value* of each new patient, by referral source, entering the practice this month?" Capturing this data is simple. Have the front desk staff print a spare copy of the patient intake form, with a space for staff to write down patient responses to a short series of marketing questions, and space for the doctors to write down the diagnosis, treatment plan, and anticipated *five year* cash flow from the new patient. (For example, an 83-year-old patient with cataracts who is just passing through your office once for a routine exam while on vacation to your community will be worth a fraction of a younger glaucoma patient who you will see longitudinally for a decade.) These individual data sheets are subsequently collated and analyzed. The results quickly reveal the real return on investment for every line item of near-term marketing expenditure. Your current computer reports probably show that a new patient from Optometrist X is worth just $125—what's posted in the system this month. Instead, that new patient, over the course of their tenure with you and with their multiple procedures and their referral of friends, may be worth tens of thousands of dollars. Which starts to substantiate stronger optometric outreach efforts.

Taking this enhanced new patient reporting approach, you may learn that a dollar invested in senior screening programs returns $10, or that distant phone book advertising is a very poor return on investment.

In your own practice, staff can perform this assessment periodically to fine-tune your marketing budget or make a regular monthly report.
Here are additional marketing research and development efforts we often recommend in client practices that you may want to consider for your own practice:

"My Mother Has Cataracts" Surveys

Call every optometric office in your service area with the following script: "My mother lives in Vermont and she's just been diagnosed with cataracts...she's going to be visiting us this summer, and she would like to get a second opinion. Who would you recommend I have her see?" Responses from the optometrists' receptionists accurately reflect referral patterns from each office. Use the resulting information, and your own internal new patient sourcing statistics, to assess your ability to establish or expand a referral network. During the same survey calls, you can also ask about where to go for LASIK surgery, which may generate an entirely different set of answers.

Secret Shopper Surveys

Hire one or more thoughtful, mock patients to make appointments and receive care. The staff and doctors should be told in advance, "Sometime in the next three months we will have three survey specialists visit the practice pretending to be patients. They will have a routine exam, experience all the things our real patients do, and then report back to us on how we did."

Service Area Mapping

One of the first things we have exceptionally competitive clients do is post a large-scale map of their entire service area in their administrators or managing partners' office, or in the board room. We then add pins for all offices, prospective new offices, competing ophthalmic providers, potential consolidation targets, hospitals and large clinics. For each office, we pull the location of last 50 new patients to enter the practice and put a pin or dot on the map for them, too. The result is a useful visual aid for consolidation discussions, and a reminder to all partners of the agreed marketing and development goals.

Patient Focus Groups

There is no faster way to gain an impression of the total eye care product you're producing than to gather a formal discussion session of 8 to 12 patients who share something in common (e.g.: all are three month cataract post-ops or refractive surgery advertising leads who have not gone forward with surgery). Compensate the participants with a small check or gift certificate. You need a quiet room, refreshments, a moderator, a video camera and an operator (or you can simply audio record the meeting). Start with a few warm-up questions going completely around the table, then get to the tough questions about what your practice needs to do better. Seniors typically take 45 minutes to warm up and give you their true feelings. Younger patients are far less reserved, and will tell you what's wrong almost from the start. This is a great forum for testing proposed advertising or finding out how to fill gaps in patient service.

Researching Your Future Medical Business Environment

There is no more valuable big-picture strategic orientation for your practice than to find out what's really happening to the health care delivery system in your community. Hold face-to-face interviews with local hospital officials, benefits managers, administrators and medical directors of any larger single or multi-specialty clinics, and provider relations managers in all local managed care entities.

Let's turn from research to tactics, and dive in by saying that everyone works better when they can follow a few simple rules. Here are six simple rules that you can apply to every one of the tactics discussed below, the tactics that work best in eye care marketing today.

Rule One

Even if your goal is a steady-state practice, have the business discipline to allocate 3 percent to 5 percent of revenue (collections) for marketing expenditures. You may need to raise this to as much as 20 percent, at least initially, if you're growing a elective-service practice like LASIK in an extremely competitive market. Don't go back and forth with your total dollar commitment, and especially avoid knee-jerk responses to your competitor's efforts. You should largely run your own race.

Rule Two

Allocate your global marketing budget to those marketing tools you believe (or experience in other settings shows) have the highest return on investment. For example, OD outreach and making calls to patients lost to follow up can have a 70:1 return. By comparison, TV cataract ads rarely perform over 5:1. When you hear about some great new tactic, always ask: "Who else has tried this? How long have they been at it? What are their verified results?"

Rule Three

Put sufficient dollars and time into each marketing tool you decide to use. A common beginner's error is to spend too little, for too short a time, get bored with your own efforts, and shift prematurely to the next marketing whim. Another error is to spread your budget thinly among too many tactics.

Rule Four

Don't think that managed care, now or in the future, removes the need for marketing. Even in a largely capitated market you still have to establish and maintain exchange relationships, not only with patients and primary care doctors, but with payer officials. Neglect of the latter, especially, can lead to profound vulnerability. Changes in the marketplace may alter your tactics, but your budget allocations and your "marketing mindset" should be unchanging.

Rule Five

Don't spend any of your budget on external marketing (eg: advertising, publicity, outreach) until you've spent sufficiently to anchor a solid base of internal marketing (customer research, staff education, facility upgrades, recall protocols, etc.)

Rule Six

Use marketing research in direct proportion to your aspirations and budget. If you can't afford the luxury of ongoing research, at least put adequate resources into a periodic but formal sampling of patient satisfaction, patient sourcing and developments of the local competitive environment.

Marketing, and particularly paid ads, can waste dollars and slaughter profits and cash flow better than any other unmonitored costs. Marketing, as every thriving ophthalmologist knows, is a key fuel for your practice vehicle. Some practices seem to need nitro-boosted dragster fuel. Others chug along just fine on charcoal.

Why do certain practices find it essential to spend 20 percent of every dollar they collect for aggressive advertising, while others spend 1 percent on little more than holiday gifts to referring doctors? There are many reasons for the vast differences, but they boil down to just these ten…try to find your practice, left or right, on the chart that follows.

Marketing Cost-Sparing Practices	Marketing High-Cost Practices
The practice has little or no competition.	The practice has significant competition.
The practice is at a volume threshold, and the doctors desire no further growth.	The practice is still being driven by its owners to grow rapidly.
The doctor's services are unchanging.	The doctors are introducing new services.
The practice has a large pool of past patients and lives on alumni referral.	The practice is young and needs to build a patient base.
The practice relies largely on physician and optometric referral; these referrals still have a finite cost, but it's lower than paid ads.	The practice is poorly supported by doctor referrals, and needs to communicate to the public for self-referring patients.
The practice does an excellent job of maintaining a long-term relationship with each patient, and therefore doesn't need as many *new* patients to feed the practice.	The practice offers poor services, or hs a faulty recall system, and therefore needs a constant stream of new patients.
The doctors would rather have the last few percent of practice profits distributed as a no-risk personal bonus, than to take the risk of "betting the bonus" for greater profits.	The doctors have significant personal spending discipline; they earn a comfortable living, and are willing to roll the dice with their retained earnings.
The practice tried the wrong kind of marketing—or the right kind of marketing for too short a timeframe—and got burned.	The practice's marketing efforts have either worked, or it's too early to tell and the doctors have the discipline to stick with it.
The doctors are economically conservative and resist taking business risks unless the outcome is fairly certain.	The doctors are willing to take calculated risks to grow the business.
The doctors are politically conservative and don't wish to stand out in the community.	The doctors are either self-confident or at least cavalier enough to not be concerned about the opinion of other physicians.

Are you and your practice at either of these extremes, or somewhere in the middle? Either extreme, of too much or too little spending, may represent poor practice management. Finding the right marketing fuel—and opening the throttle to the right burn rate—is an essential ongoing business exercise.

As a first step in the assessment of your situation, prepare a graph for the past 12-18 months of the number of month-by-month new and total patient visits in the practice. In multi-doctor practices, have a separate graph for each doctor. In practices with multiple offices, sort the data by location and prepare graphs for each office, as well.

With these graphs and your practice's financials on hand as a reference, let's now discuss the norms, and how this can influence your ad budget.

In a general ophthalmology practice, it's normal to spend about 3 percent to 8 percent of collections on the total marketing function (excluding internal staff costs such as telemarketers or screeners). An old-line, established practice with no further growth aspirations and a kind market environment may get by on 1 percent or 2 percent. New practices, elective care surgeons and surgeons in overserved, competitive markets may need to spend much, much more.

Back to your new and total patient graphs, which may look something like the graphs below:

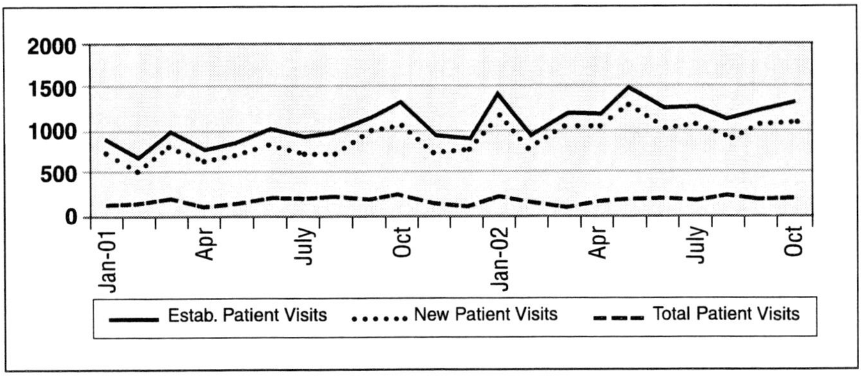

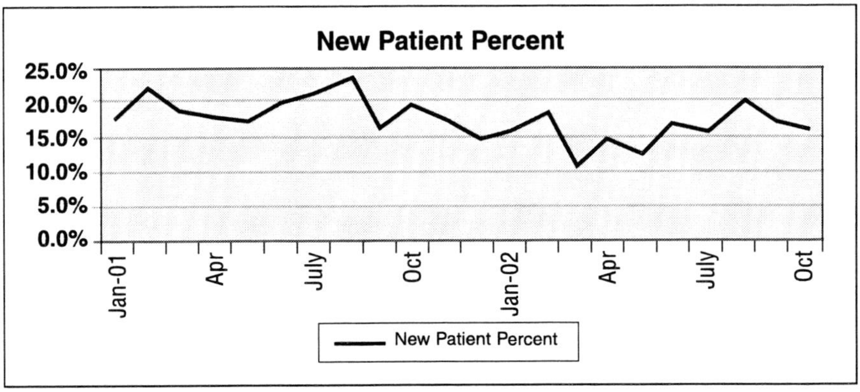

New patients in a general practice should represent 10 to 20 percent of total visits. This can and should range somewhat higher in a subspecialty or referral-based practice. Younger satellite offices will obviously have a much higher ratio of new patients. Higher percentages than this baseline for an established practice may indicate poor continuity of care and recall protocols, which should be audited for gaps.

The existing and desired surgical density of the practice is another key driver for marketing budgets. In a typical general ophthalmology practice, it's normal to transit +/-25 total patient visits (including post ops) for every cataract surgery case performed. A higher number of total visits per surgical case may mean there are too few *new* patients to feed the surgical schedule, and the practice is providing routine care over and over again to the same patients. Each surgeon should examine their case selection criteria and, if warranted, consider a more aggressive approach. Or if you find your care selection criteria (even if conservative) to be appropriate, you may be placed in a position of having to market more than the average doctor to generate a desired case volume.

The most important single determinant of how much—and how—you spend on marketing should be the desired mix and number of new patients. On the advertising side of a total marketing program, we know from experience that it can take from $50 to $500 to generate a new patient lead (and even more than this for a single surgical case) depending on the market, the service promoted and the branding that's been established.

Every doctor within your practice should declare and frequently update their volume performance goals so that the total marketing budget walks in lock step with the composite goals of the overall practice. Nothing smokes out a practice's strategic conflict faster than when we get the entire management and doctor team together in one room and point out that the doctors are asking for 100 new surgical cases a month—immediately—but only giving marketing the resources for 10. Marketing, perhaps like farming, is a long-range activity, best done with patience, long-term planning and crossed fingers. Any need to ramp up the practice's patient flow should be anticipated as far in advance as possible, because the lag time from conception to execution to impact can be many quarters or even a matter of years.

To help make the need for marketing less of an emergency and more planned, it may help to install an early warning system in your practice. Each month look forward 90 days out in the clinic and surgical schedule, and plot the number of patient visits and surgical cases currently scheduled on a month-by-month graph. This forward-looking trend data will at least give you a little more time to react, and may keep you from over-shooting or under-shooting what's needed to keep the practice growing. Of equal value, it will keep the doctors from panicking every time there's a lull in the surgical schedule if they can see a repeating seasonal pattern each year.

Marketing, as a department within your practice and as a business discipline, is annoyingly resistant to cost-benefit analysis. The old saw is dead on: "I know that half of my marketing budget is wasted…I just don't know which half." Experience has shown that we can perhaps decrease the "wasted" factor to 25 percent or less if we stick to activities shown empirically in other settings to work well. The premium you pay to be able to use syndicated marketing materials proven effective in other markets can be far less expensive than inventing the wheel yourself. For an established, somewhat more vanguard than average general practice, performing a mix of cataract and refractive surgery, here's a reasonable budget apportionment:

- The first marketing dollars spent, representing 10 percent or more of the annual budget should be spent internally, on everything from patient education literature to a looped video on your services in the waiting room. Special attention should be spent on getting recall protocols up to "zero defects," and having the doctors and staff actively asking each patient for referrals.

- If your practice is dependent on optometry referrals (or wants to be), the next dollars spent, perhaps another 10 percent, should be on outreach efforts, which can include personal visits, continuing education sessions, part-time facility rental agreements, and other network development.

- For practices oriented to senior eye care, external screening programs are next in line for return on investment, and deserve perhaps the next 5-10 percent slice of the marketing pie.

- The heavy, external lifting needs to be borne by paid advertising, which for this specimen practice should probably consume up to 60 percent or more of the total marketing budget. The apportionment to creative and production, as compared to media is highly dependent on the situation. In principle, however, don't blow all of your budget on creating great advertising, and then only have a little left over to publish or air your ads. That would be like spending all of your budget on a great car, and then not having enough money left over to buy gas.

- Supplemental external marketing should include about 5 percent of the budget spent on formal efforts to generate publicity; using your hospital's house publicist as the conduit to the working press can spare costs.

- Hold 10 to 15 percent of any budget in reserve for oversight and for rotating exploratory efforts. For example, a LASIK practice using radio and print only, should test TV infomercials next, a formal sales training course, or a corporate outreach program. Any of these experiments found to work better than what you have done in the past deserves an enduring portion of the overall marketing budget and should displace an under-performing tactic.

- It should go without saying that a practice of any marketing sophistication at all already has a formal protocol for thanking referral sources through calls, cards, letters and small gifts, the cost of which is trivial on a cost-per-lead basis when compared with paid advertising. (Indeed, if patient-to-patient referral is not stimulated side-by-side with a media advertising program, the practice is likely going to tread water or drown, because costly advertised leads often only break even…it's the derivative alumni referrals that start being profitable.)

- To the extent possible, every prospective patient calling the practice, and every new patient actually entering the practice should be tracked. Trends should be noted, and there should be a feedback loop between the weekly or monthly cost-per-lead statistics and the marketing mix. Specific tactics and media shown by the numbers to be under performing should be continuously flushed from the program.

You can tell from the language of marketing that we still have a lot to learn. Disappointments are managed and faces saved by calling a failed marketing effort an "experiment" or "an investment in the future." As you sign all those big checks that pay for your marketing program, track the numbers, and you'll feel a little better about the level of control you have over what will always remain one of the most vexing and mysterious business challenges in you practice.

Because ad content tends to raise the most client questions, let's now discuss what works best.

First, comes branding—the heart of which is the name of the company. What should your practice's name be? Here are a few guidelines. Your name should describe what you do: Smith Eye Clinic is obviously better than Smith Clinic. It should have no more than three words, four at the most, if possible: "Smith Eye Associates of the Southwest" is little cumbersome. Avoid using a geographic identifier if this is over-used in your service area "Cumberland Eye Care." Avoid a name that boxes you in geographically or in the services you provide. If you live in a twin-cities area, don't name your practice after just one city. If you are going to offer total eye care, don't name your practice "The Eye Surgery Center." A personalized practice name can be extremely effective. And Dr. Smith, his staff and patients are perhaps going to have more pride going to "Smith Eye Care" than something more generic. However, what happens when Dr. Smith tries to take on an associate? Unless the second doctor is very subordinate, he or she can be understandably demoralized laboring in the founder's shadow. A proper name is memorable for branding purposes, and that's really the important concept to remember.

Second comes the matter of graphic standards and image development. Consistency, even more than elegance, is the key. Can your practice's graphic design work pass this test? Take one copy of all your print ads, your stationary, your brochures, signage, etc. Mount them on the wall and step back 30 feet. Does everything look like it comes from the same company? To develop a more cohesive look, have your graphic artist prepare a standards summary that describes the colors, sizes and fonts you use, the relationship of graphic elements, and the person in your practice who will approve everything going forward. Depending on how important style is to your practice (vital for refractive surgery advertisers, less so for established geriatric practices), schedule the replacement of any materials that don't fit your new standards.

Next, remember that your doctors are the product. It works best if you show your potential customers what they're buying. This pearl is overlooked by a majority of eye care advertisers. A doctor's photo with a brief bio as a caption should be included with all print ads. Radio and TV should showcase the doctor as "star" of the practice. Doing this can as much as double response rates—which should overcome any resistance you have to appearing in your own ads on the grounds that it's undignified.

Last, be sure to use patient testimonials in your advertising, which, like using the doctor's voice and image, can double response rates. Beware prohibitions in a handful of states against this, although some of these barriers have recently fallen.

Many of America's largest, most profitable and most successful eye care practices have gotten that way through their cordial relations with the optometric community which is, of course, a kind of marketing.

Independent and chain optometry practices control the distribution of eye care to the majority of commercial-aged patients and an important minority of seniors. Surgeons have been tapping into this distribution channel for decades. The historic grudging acceptance of referrals from optometrists has shifted in the last decade to relatively high levels of camaraderie, as both O's have come to realize the financial and patient care benefits of working together. Regulatory question marks may loom over these relationships in the future, but at present, warranted, ethical sharing of patients and financial reciprocity through co-management fees appear to be here to stay.

Having an optometric director is a core success factor in higher-volume referral centers, and has been the "secret weapon" of corporate co-management centers. Hiring a highly experienced center director is expensive—$120,000 and up in many cases—but could be the critical gap in your own program.

Over-dependency on a single lay staff member or optometric director for outreach can leave a practice highly vulnerable. It's critical for physician-principals to maintain a minimum threshold of direct personal contact with "key accounts."

Staff-to-staff outreach can be an effective adjunct to doctor-to-doctor contact. Your office can provide a billing help-line, develop a tech training workshop, and hold a periodic, staff-invited open house. The proliferation of competing CE programs for optometrists, in the wake of therapeutics legislation, is making these programs somewhat less effective as an outreach tool in some urban settings. Consider more personalized, in-office mini-fellowships. Provide your optometric and primary physician colleagues with referral pads, indicating the patient's name, consultation sought, appointment scheduling information and a map showing how to get to your office. Consider a private, priority doctor's hotline and designate one staffer as a chief contact. Identify, by doctor, their preferred follow-up communication (a call vs. a letter vs. a fax, etc.).

Some of the most advanced practices, including practices that were the first to co-manage with optometrists, are making a transition from purely informal and voluntary referrals to deeper business relationships. Those vanguard surgeons in the future who take their voluntary referral relationships with ODs to the end-game of merger and acquisition can expect to substantially lock up their markets and be better prepared for the next developments in managed care and cost containment.

Pro or con, every practicing surgeon, it seems, has an opinion about medical marketing. Polarization on this issue will continue and intensify. You can safely wager that whatever extremes are reached in ambulatory health care promotion, we're going to eventually see it tried first in ophthalmology.

As fees and profit margins continue to fall, and incremental volume becomes so critical, some of the nation's most ambitious providers may give P.T. Barnum a run for his money…or even Tom Mix, that other famous American promotional hound dog. Mix, a celebrated cowboy movie star of the early 20th Century, has his Rolls Royce outfitted with a pair of horns as a radiator cap, and specially molded rubber tires that imprinted his initials "TM" on the dusty roads of pre-pavement Hollywood. If elite diamond merchant deBeers now lasers their logo on diamonds, can we be that far away from a time with eye surgeons looking for an edge will micro-tattoo their logos on the eyes of willing patients? Only the future will tell.

Chapter Twelve: Reducing the Risk of Not Being Paid By HMOs and IPAs

By Richard E. Gable, PhD, MBA

Ophthalmologists and optometrists around the country are experiencing a common problem: HMO's, insurance companies, and Independent Practice Associations (IPAs) are not paying legitimate claims for services rendered. The disturbing trend includes:

- Unjustified denial of claims
- Repeated requests for additional claims
- Delays in payment
- Reduction in payment
- No payment at all because the third party payer has gone bankrupt

In my experience, once a payer gets into financial trouble, ophthalmologists have very limited options for recovering their unpaid fees. To reduce the risk of not getting paid in full, physicians need to do two things: First, investigate the HMO, insurance company, or IPA before signing a contract; and second, carefully review and negotiate the terms of the proposed contract.

Carefully Check Out The Payer

The first line of defense is to learn what you can about the party with whom you propose to sign a contract. Among other things, you should ask and get answers to the following questions:

1. How many years has the payer been in business? Generally the more years the better.
2. What is the payer's marketshare and who is its competition? The more dominate the payer the less likely it will go bankrupt.
3. Has the payer had recent rapid growth through mergers and acquisitions?

4. What is the payer's record of paying claims fully, accurately, and on time? Ask other ophthalmologists and medical groups for their experience with the payer.

5. If you contract with an IPA, does it have adequate funds on hand for incurred but not reported claims (IBNRs)? If not, this could be a warning sign of inadequate capitalization and financial control.

6. What are the background, experience, and track record of key officers and management? If an outside company manages the IPA, what is the management company's track record?

How do you get answers to these questions? A good way to begin is by checking the payer's financial statements. These may be on file with your State Department of Insurance or, if a publicly traded company, with the Federal Securities and Exchange Commission. You can also ask the payer to provide you with its most recent financial statements. Other valuable sources of information include your colleagues and local, state, and national medical and group practice associations. Healthcare attorneys and consultants may also have useful, first hand information about the payer.

Negotiating The Contract

Even if a background check does not reveal any obvious problems, physicians still need to carefully negotiate the terms of their provider agreements with HMOs, insurance companies, and IPAs. Physicians often feel that these contracts are presented on a "take it or leave it" basis. Although this is sometimes true, in most cases, important changes can be made. The key is to know what to ask for and what to avoid. Among the negotiating points you should consider are the following:

1. No contract is better than a bad contract;

2. It may be preferable to contract with multiple payers rather than have a single payer account for a substantial portion of your managed care business;

3. Any promises that have been made orally or in preliminary correspondence (example – to carve out certain services from your scope of responsibility, risk pool participation, and exclusivity) must be included in the final written agreement;

4. You should have the right to receive financial information about the payer on an ongoing basis, such as quarterly;

5. You should have the right to audit the payer's books and records to determine whether you are being paid accurately;

6. If you are paid under capitation, the contract should state exactly what services you will be expected to perform for this fixed fee. Preferably, the service matrix should be detailed by CPT code. It is not enough to say, for example, that you are broadly responsible for "ophthalmology services;"
7. Avoid contract terms that allow the payer to unilaterally change the scope of services for which you are responsible;
8. All key terms (such as "medically necessary" and "emergency") should be clearly defined;
9. If you are to be paid pursuant to a fee schedule, is the fee schedule attached?; and
10. If there is a reference to an outside fee schedule, such as Medicare rates, do you fully understand what those rates are?

Post-termination rates need to be addressed for patients who you may be required to continue to treat for some period after the contract ends. You should avoid provisions that allow the payer to penalize you for failure to comply with the payer's policy and procedures or that allow the payer to unilaterally reduce your rate of compensation because of the payer's financial difficulties or for any other reason. The contract should be specific about when you will be paid. Will it be based upon calendar days or working days? Most states now have in effect "prompt payment" laws; however, the enforcement of these laws has been spotty. Therefore, you want to make sure that your contract is explicit on this important point. Be careful about provisions that require payment only after a" clean claim" is submitted. The chief reason payers use to justify non-payment is that allegedly the claim is not clean. Therefore, what constitutes a clean claim needs to be clearly defined.

Be on the lookout for hidden provisions that require you to appeal claim denials within a short time such as 30-60 days. If you fail to appeal within the time specified, your claim will be barred. Either these "contractual statutes of limitations" should be eliminated or the appeals period should be significantly increased.

Try to secure the right to retain payment from any secondary payers at least up to the level of your bill charges. If you will not be able to retain "coordination of benefits" payments, then you should reduce or eliminate any obligations to assist the payer to collect such payments.

Watch out for "all products provisions." Some contracts may oblige you to provide discounts to the payer other than those expressly covered in the contract you signed. Indeed, you may inadvertently end up giving the PPO discount you approved to the payer's indemnity insurance patients. Even worse, you may be providing discounts to payers with whom you are not even contracted so called "silent PPOs"! A number of states (e.g. Alaska, Kentucky, Maryland, Massachusetts, Nevada, and Texas) have made such provisions illegal.

If you are paid by capitation, you should limit their retroactive dis-enrollment to no more than 90 days. Furthermore, if you actually provide services to a patient who is later determined to have been ineligible and you cannot collect from the patient after two billing cycles, then the payer should be required to pay you on a previously agreed upon fee for service basis.

If you are eligible to participate in risk pool distributions, the contract needs to define your rights clearly. It is preferable to get payments on a quarterly rather than an annual basis. You should also try to get the payer to segregate the risk pool money and not co-mingle it with the payer's other funds.

If possible, try to negotiate for the maintenance of a security deposit equal to one to two months of capitation. If a security deposit is established, then you want to be given a security interest on the money. In the event that the payer goes bankrupt, you will then have the right to the money, which will not be included in the assets to be used to pay the general creditors.

The contract language should have a provision that you can terminate the contract for non-payment. Try to keep the time period the payer has to attempt to remedy a breech of contract for non-payment as short as possible; ten days, for example, is obviously preferable to the 30-60 days typically allowed to correct other types of breaches. You should also have the right to terminate for chronic late payment.

The contract should provide that your attorney's fees will be paid in the event you have to sue or arbitrate to get paid. You should avoid contract requirements for extended, non-binding mediation periods. Arbitration may allow you to collect unpaid claims more quickly and at less cost than if you had to go to court. You should avoid provisions that require you to make an arbitration demand within a shorter time than the statue of limitations for a breech of contract. An arbitration provision should provide for broad discovery rights, a neutral arbitrator, and a location convenient to you and not at the payer's out-of-state headquarters.

Be sure to avoid contract provisions that allow the payer to amend the contract without your consent. Similarly, watch out for contract provisions that incorporate the payer's policies and procedures that may be inconsistent with the contract.

Finally, the contract should provide that when it terminates, your post-termination care obligations will be limited to a reasonable period of time while your patients decide whether to find another physician. You should also carefully review non-solicitation provisions to be sure that they do not unfairly restrict your ability to contact the patients in the event of termination.

The old adage "an ounce of prevention is worth a pound of cure" certainly applies to managed care contracts. By carefully checking out with whom you are contracting, and then negotiating a fair contract that protects your interests, you can significantly reduce your risk of not being paid.

What's the next step after the managed care contract has been executed? Organizing managed care operations. Recommendations for delineating key rolls and responsibilities and using information systems to support managed care operations are a mandate in today's marketplace.

Third Party Administration Recommendations

The practice needs to develop third party administrative protocols to create cohesive working relationships between the front desk, checkout, surgery scheduler, and billing/collections staff. I would recommend the following:

1. The practice should assign an individual to coordinate the managed care contracting process. The MC Coordinator should serve as the community liaison with the various managed care plans, medical groups, IPAs, health systems, capitated ophthalmology networks, and academic centers;
2. This individual should be assigned to work under the supervision of the administrator who would be responsible to complete the managed care provider applications and take care of the physician credentialing process. This individual should take the initiative to red flag the executed contracts 120 days prior to their annual renewal term so the practice has ample time to prepare should they decide to renegotiate the contract; and
3. The practice should develop a managed care reference manual for the front desk and billing departments. This managed care resource should contain the following data:
    - Primary care physician preauthorization guidelines;
    - HMO member eligibility department contact and phone number;
    - Coordination of benefits contact and phone number;
    - At which hospital must the surgical procedures be performed?;
    - Emergency services guidelines;
    - Reimbursement methodology and rates;

- Co-payment amounts;
- Billing procedures and timeline for billing;
- Payment turnaround time; and
- Special utilization management protocols such as surgical second opinion program, hospital precertification, etc.

4. You need to develop an administrative procedure to identify when the various managed care contracts come up for renewal. The practice needs adequate time to profile the contracts from a plan compliance and profitability perspective. The contract renegotiation process needs to begin at least 120 days prior to the annual anniversary date. All managed care contracts have language that stipulate the contract will automatically renew at the original reimbursement rates and terms unless renegotiated.

5. The practice should develop a methodology to identify the newsletters that are sent out by managed care plans informing practices of plan changes, new billing procedures and other administrative changes necessary to remain in compliance with the contract terms. The practice should develop interoffice communication procedures to make sure that the information is disseminated to the appropriate satellite offices to insure continuity of administrative services.

6. I recommend that your practice contact the provider relation's coordinator to schedule an orientation session for the billing and front desk personnel whenever your practice enters into a new managed care contract.

7. Practices need to develop administrative follow-up protocols to make sure the practice is listed in the HMO/PPO provider and member directories. It is not uncommon for providers in a given community to be excluded from the published directories. The managed care organizations publish the directory annually and then on an as-need basis. Your practice will need to identify the individual in the provider relations department responsible for maintaining current provider and member directories. The provider relation's representative will be able to provide the practice with the necessary information to make sure that your practice is included in the next publication. The practice needs to specify to the managed care plans that they expect all your office locations to be included in the publication. Most managed care plans will only list the primary office unless instructed otherwise.

8. Your practice will eventually be required to develop a patient satisfaction instrument and conduct periodic exit interviews and/or mail out survey instruments so that they can measure the patients' perception of their experience at your practice. The managed care industry is now tying financial incentives and disincentives to patient feedback regarding their level of satisfaction with the medical services received at a contracted providers office.

9. Managed care contracts should be viewed as individual profit centers for your practice. The practice should evaluate the revenues generated on a contract-by-contract basis to determine if the managed care plan fulfilled their promised financial and patient business development goals. Practices should always measure what percentage of the practice's total annual revenues did the individual managed care contract generate. Managed care marketing strategies should be created by payer type (HMO versus PPO) to systematically increase the annual revenues per managed care contract year to year. How many of your referral sources know what managed care plans you participate in?

Conclusion

Physicians are trained as scientists. Therefore, they are accustomed to making decisions based upon pertinent information. So, it is not surprising that when faced with standard managed care contracts, physicians want to do more than sign on the dotted line. "Do more" usually means turning to the reimbursements schedule before deciding to sign. But the sections of the contract dealing with how managed care organizations administer its product and program, is often overlooked, which is of equal importance.

This managed care chapter was developed to address the needs that many physicians have expressed for guidance in contracts evaluation, negotiating agreements, and how to effectively administer the contracts to insure maximum profitability.

I have tried to provide an overview of the issues involved in managed care contracting and offer practical ways for physicians to effectively operate in a managed care environment. While this chapter cannot entirely replace the specific advice physicians should seek from attorneys and other experts, it can help doctors take their place at the negotiating table across from managed care executives with greater authority and confidence.

Chapter Thirteen:
Improving Practice Cash Flow by Adding Partner Doctors and Keeping Them Happy and Productive

A surprisingly high percentage of ophthalmologists are still in solo practice, most quite happily. On the plus side, solo practice provides the satisfaction and serenity of absolute control. Solo surgeons don't have to consult with a colleague. They don't have to confront peers on difficult business or medical issues—they need only face down subordinates.

Soloists can spend the company's profits as they see fit...the only financial negotiations are between the doctor, their administrator, and their spouse. Soloists can come and go as they please. Meetings are pared to a bare minimum. "Absolute bliss," some surgeons might say.

"Bliss" is not a word that comes readily to mind with a majority of doctors in group practice, that more commonly find themselves in a marriage of convenience. And for at least *some* doctors in *some* groups, two, three or more doctors working together are not so much a trim commando squad as an armed gang, as likely to turn on each other as rumble with the local competition. Still, the economic and professional advantages of group practice are compelling, and may trump your desire for independence; in the same way that for most adults the trials of married life are better than the trials of being single.

There are many practical advantages of group practice. The foremost is financial. One of the best ways for a busy, growing soloist to improve personal profits is to add a second doctor. Unfortunately, the founding doctor can be too penny-pinching, limiting the choice of associates to those at the bottom of the pack. A more generous approach can be more profitable to the senior doctor in the long run. Founding doctors often overlook that profit gains arise more from fixed overhead sharing on their own side, than from passive income flowing from a grab at the new doctor's profits. Here are sample numbers pointing this out:

	Solo/Founder Doctor Before Hiring a Second Doctor	Two Doctor Practice
Founding Doctor Collections	$1,000,000	$900,000
New Doctor Collections	0	600,000
Total Collections	1,000,000	1,500,000
Fixed Expenses (expenses that don't materially change based on variations in practice volume between one and two doctors...eg: rent, utilities, accounting, core staff, office management, etc.)	360,000	360,000
Variable Expenses (those that rise in lockstep with increased patient volume...eg: medical supplies, tech staffing, etc.)	240,000	340,000
New Doctor Compensation	0	200,000
Total Expenses	600,000	900,000
Profit Available for Founding Doctor	$400,000	$600,000

As you can see from this very simplified example, even if the founding doctor's practice is mildly cannibalized by the new doctor's arrival, he takes a net pay increase. In this case, he produces 10 percent less, but gets a 50 percent pay raise, which is still more than substantiated by the financial risks of adding a doctor and the stresses of managing a larger office and a fellow professional.

There are numerous other advantages of growing into a larger practice. Expensive technology upgrades can be shared, potentially increasing the quality of care. Keeping in mind that a significant proportion of new technology is quickly obsolesced, the pain of buying errors can be split up. The quality of care may be higher in group practices for two other reasons. First, because surgeons can obviously learn from their peers, especially if periodic case reviews and chart audits are conducted. Second, because two or more surgeons working together represent a kind of internal oversight, even if there is no formal case review process.

Patients can be better served if several sub-specialists are present. Care is better coordinated, more convenient and a patient's needs can all be addressed in a single location. Doctors in solo practices often report that they feel somewhat isolated professionally. The difference between being a group or solo doctor is a little like the difference between playing tennis with a partner across the net or whacking the ball against your garage door. The physical motions are about the same, but the game can be more interesting and the learning curve is much steeper, if you play with someone. With a partner, you have someone with whom you can share successes and commiserate failures.

It's much easier to afford superior management talent, along with top-flight accountants, attorneys, consultants, and other advisors if their cost is borne by several doctors working together. Let's say you need an attorney to review and negotiate your new building lease. This will cost in the range of a few hundred to a few thousand dollars, depending on the complexities. It takes just about as much time to negotiate terms on a 2,500 square foot space for a soloist and the 8,000 square foot space for three doctors.

As a member of a group practice, you have an in-house sounding board to help you improve your good ideas, and a safety check to help you avoid following through with poor ideas. (An ideal combination is when one surgeon is oriented to cost containment, and his or her partner is oriented to revenue-enhancement.).

There is greater practice security. When a solo surgeon falls ill, the practice grinds to an immediate halt. A second or third surgeon can keep the company going until the downed partner is back in action. This especially critical when your practice includes an ambulatory surgery center, with high fixed costs.

On the subject of ASC's and other ancillaries, adding a doctor to your practice (or simply merging practices) can substantiate the development of these side business lines that one doctor's surgical volume could not support. A doctor who performs 30 cataracts a months cannot support a surgery center. Two doctors that do 60 cases <u>between</u> them can develop an ASC that generates $200,000 or more in profits per year. In the typical settings, that's a 30 percent or greater pay raise for each doctor, and a better surgical environment, for virtually no extra personal work once the facility is up and running.

There can be significant lifestyle benefits, as well. Call coverage is shared. It's even possible to arrange periodic sabbaticals, giving each doctor a block of several weeks off every year, or even months off every few years. Two part-time surgeons can job-share.

Many soloists we consult with are unsure about the timing of adding the second doctor to the practice. It's critical to forecast the almost inevitable cash flow crunch that occurs early on as you take on a new associate or partner and to have both the patience and the cash reserves to take a personal pay cut for several quarters or longer.

Let's imagine a solo surgeon with $1.2 million in revenue and a 40 percent profit margin. Near term, especially if there are delays in gaining licensure or panel status, the new associate will represent all outgo and no income. It's typical for a general ophthalmologist-associate's first year costs (including wages, taxes, benefits, relocation costs, insurance, staffing and other professional support) to reach $250,000 or more. In the early months, there will be sharp drops in practice profit, and the senior doctor has no recourse except to reduce his salary or draw on loan proceeds to preserve his income. The table below shows a typical, if markedly simplified and somewhat accelerated, cash flow in the first several months.

	Base Month	Month 1	2	3	4	5	6
Number of MDs	1	2	2	2	2	2	2
Base Collections	100000	100000	100000	100000	100000	100000	100000
New doctor collections	0	8000	15000	25000	30000	35000	40000
Total collections	100000	108000	115000	125000	130000	135000	140000
Base Expenses	60000	60000	60000	60000	60000	60000	60000
New doctor expenses, including salaries	0	25000	22000	20000	18000	18000	18000
Total expenses	60000	85000	82000	80000	78000	78000	78000
Profit for senior doctor	40000	23000	33000	45000	52000	57000	62000

As you can see from this highly stylized example, if the new doctor's productivity can be accelerated (as by pre-arrival marketing, strong outreach efforts, banking cases for subspecialists, etc.), the senior doctor has only a short-term drop in personal income, followed by a very sharp increase. Obviously, you don't want to stretch out the process. A senior doctor who earns $40,000 in the base month before a new hire's arrival is going to resent the young colleague who becomes stuck at a "month 2" level of productivity, which would result in a significant and durable income drop for the senior doctor.

For the same reason, you also don't want to bring a new doctor on prematurely. Here are a few rules of thumb:

1. Before you bring on a new doctor to form a two-doctor general ophthalmology practice, you should personally see <u>at least</u> 20 percent more patients per month than you can comfortably fit into your schedule. This typically translates to 600 or more patient visits per month for a general ophthalmologist

(inclusive of paid as well as post op visits.) Alternately, you should have reached (but not yet exceeded) your comfortable personal patients volumes, be growing total patient volumes at least 10 percent a year, and have a high level of confidence that this growth rate will continue along with a higher level of financial reserves to carry the new doctor.

2. This level of excess productivity (or superior growth rate) should have been in place for at least the last six months before you make a hiring commitment. From this, you can see that it's occasionally appropriate to begin the doctor search process before you think you actually might need additional help, especially if you work in a less-desirable market. It may take 12-24 months or more to find a superior candidate in such settings.
3. Make sure you have significant financial reserves in place to carry you through the first few soft quarters after your new doctor arrives. Whether these reserves are held as retained earnings of the practice, personal savings or simply a line of credit, you should have access to the equivalent of not less that six times your monthly salary and draws. Also, be prepared to curtail personal lifestyle costs temporarily if your new doctor takes a little longer than expected to build his or her practice.

Once you have transitioned from one doctor to two, the fastest way to murder both cash flow and professional satisfaction in your practice is to have an unfruitful union. Your new favorite saying has to become, "I can live with that."

If you are married and find it quite difficult to live with your real-life spouse, the odds go up in our experience that you may find the same challenges in your business "marriage." Conversely, if you enjoy a harmonious marriage with your family spouse, you can successfully apply the same tactics that work here to your business marriage. Even though you're the senior doctor, take pains to ask your new partner or partner-to-be what they think about new practice initiatives or expenditures. Like an ex-bachelor, you can no longer do the ophthalmic equivalent of staying out late (not coming in on time for work), hanging out with friends (running behind in clinic), or spending money freely (buying a new laser without asking permission first.)

You should accept that bringing on a fellow doctor and becoming a small group practice will involve more than just near-term financial pain. Longer-term, there will be other discomforts. Chief among these, additional meeting and communication time is essential. Here's the minimum line-up for real success:

- If you don't already hold general staff meetings, these should be conducted at least every two months; monthly is preferable. All doctors should be in attendance.

- If the practice is up to a size suggesting departmentalization, department meetings should be held monthly; at least one doctor should attend at least every other technical department meeting.
- There should be a monthly finance and volume performance meeting with the practice manager or administrator, with all partner and partner-track doctors in attendance.
- The doctors should meet alone at least once a month. In the early months, and perhaps durably, the doctors should review a cross-section of random charts to compare care pathways, referral patterns (both intra- and inter-practice), return intervals and utilization.
- Depending on everyone's temperament, it's a nice touch to arrange a social meeting of the doctors every quarter or two. These meetings are most often dinners or similar outings with spouses; beyond mere enjoyment, they serve to deepen the bonds between partners. Please keep in mind that these social ties are not essential. There is no absolute requirement that doctors in a group be buddies in their private lives; indeed, too much personal involvement can cloud business judgment and create the opportunity for a personal spat (or worse, a spouse-to-spouse argument) to spill over into the business.

In the vast majority of cases, as you make the transition from a solo to two-doctor or larger practice, your new doctor will spend two to three preliminary years as a partner-track associate. During this trial period, he or she should receive their personal monthly production figures (patient visits, surgical cases, collections and average revenue yield per patient visit); ideally, these are graphed to make it easier to spot trends. In addition, we feel strongly that partner-track associates in good standing should receive some or all of the financial performance statistics for the overall practice. Unfortunately, some senior doctors elect to keep practice financials a secret until the associate is about to become a partner. This commonly results in an associate who is untrusting, disengaged from the details of the practice, and unfit to assume the fiduciary role of a partner or company officer.

As the senior doctor, you should foster an environment of strategic intimacy. You and your new doctor should openly discuss where you want to take the practice in the future, just as young couples discuss how many children they want to raise, and what kind of home they dream of owning together. In our experience, the second greatest source of partner discord, after financial squabbles, is when doctors disagree on where the practice is heading strategically. Ideally, you and your colleague/s should collaborate on a written plan that includes:

- The geographic span of the practice (the boundaries of your service area.)
- The agreed scope of practice services and positioning strategy (eg: will you be known as a full-service provider, or a cataract boutique?)
- The provider mix (how many surgeons? Medical ophthalmologists? ODs?)
- Your current and future financial performance, out at least five years. This section of your strategic summary should describe if your developmental bias will be toward high market share (which will likely constrain profit margins) or high profit margins (which will likely constrain market share.)

For real development of your associate, make sure the associate has non-clinical as well as clinical duties. Every doctor, even durable associates who are not on a partner track, should have five or more hours per month that they devote to staff education, outreach in the community, outcomes research, protocol writing, etc. Every doctor should periodically sit on various management committees and task forces.

Give your new associate reasonable control over their professional environment. It can be very helpful to give each doctor in a group a dedicated lead or primary technician. While every practice needs a degree of uniformity and standards, make sure you provide your doctor with a chance to customize certain forms and protocols, especially those germane to their subspecialty expertise. Don't force your associate to adopt your surgical approach and don't impose yourself as an uninvited proctor. Presumably you have selected your new colleague wisely, and respect this doctor's existing personality, skills, and professional judgment. Like love and marriage, don't hold out hope that you're going to be able to change your partner-to-be, even if they promise to change.

Disclose early on, ideally when the initial contract is signed, what the buy-in terms are going to be for partner-track associates. We most often advise clients to spell out *provisional, non-binding* terms in writing as part of the initial employment agreement. These terms should include a) when a partnership opportunity is likely to be first offered, b) what segments of the practice will be sold (eg: will ASC shares be offered, or just shares in the professional corporation), c) what percent may be offered, d) how the practice will be valued, and e) whether financing for the buy-in will be carried by the practice or by a third-party lender.
In talking to hundreds of associate and partners doctors every year it's clear most of them are "mostly" happy. Those who aren't rank their chief complaints in the following approximate order:

1. "I don't really ever feel appreciated here; I feel like second fiddle." Go overboard in expressing your appreciation for your associate, and later, for your partner.

2. "I don't have enough voice in operations; I'm never consulted." Obviously, your partner-track associate and even your minority partner have little or no legal control over the practice. But the wise senior doctor picks associates whose counsel they respect, accept, and often implement.

3. "The senior doctor gets all the cases; I'm not being fed patients, but instead have to fight for every new patient. The front desk knows who signs their paychecks, and so the senior doctor gets most of the best new patients, while I get the scraps"... Very few young associates are self-starters—they arrive on the job expecting to be fed, at least to some degree. This is solved simply with a written protocol for the entire office staff outlining how new and established patients are assigned. You can go further with consumer advertising to directly support your new doctor, and coaching help to get him pushed out and introduced in the community.

4. "Every decision my doctor-boss makes seems to be made with his personal benefit in mind. I don't trust him to make decisions that will be fair for all concerned." This complaint is a little touchier to deal with, because it involves the core personality of the senior doctor. The best surgeons tend to have the greatest difficulties in this area. We find that insight counseling for the senior doctor, combined with open discussion, lots of doctor-to-doctor face time, ongoing coaching for the senior doctor and checking in regularly for associate doctor perceptions gets the job done best. Even after near-term improvements are made, ongoing vigilance is essential to check the inevitable backsliding.

5. "Issues build up here without every being discussed." The reason for this is the common observation that most surgeons despise confrontation, and harbor fears that a small confrontation will lead to an unpleasant, all-out battle. The solution includes sufficient meeting time to air out issues, and the involvement of a third party in selected doctor meetings (such as a strong administrator) to referee disagreements and gently bend the doctors toward an intelligent consensus on the most difficult issues.

In an average year, we spend hundreds of hours constructing, deconstructing, and patching up doctor-to-doctor partnerships. At the surface, there are scores of hot-button issues that make partnerships so difficult to make and keep happy. But at deeper levels, there is perhaps just one core attribute, the degree of partner equality.

Not that *inequality* is bad. Extremely strong business partnerships (and for that matter, other kinds of partnerships like marriage) exist where both sides agree who is going to lead and who is going to follow. But the most extraordinary environ ments for surgeons to work in are often those where equality prevails.

What is a partner, really? Here's a dictionary definition that's suitable for most competitive ophthalmic environments: "A partner is one of two or more people who play together in a game against an opposing side." A drier, more legalistic definition is, "A partner is someone involved in a close, cooperating relationship with others, regulated by mutual rights and responsibilities, to further a common enterprise."

All English lessons and legal jargon aside, ophthalmic partnerships fall into two very broad and profoundly different categories.

<u>Unequal</u> Partnerships: It should be no surprise that this is the most common form of partnership, in eye care and elsewhere. Even if partners are legally and economically equal, they are rarely equal in actuality. An examination of the typical ophthalmology practice reveals a rank order of leaders and followers. The hierarchy is most commonly along lines of tenure (who came first?), economic production (who collects the most?) or natural leadership (who by raw personality is granted the most authority?) In these kinds of partnerships, decisions, and resource allocations are lopsided. The senior doctors get the choice mid-week, morning hours in the practice's surgery center; the junior doctors get Friday afternoons. The seniors get their pick of the best technicians; the juniors by default run the tech training program. The seniors are excused from call sharing; the juniors are excused from a sound night's sleep. Not a bad arrangement, if you're a senior. So long as everyone gets to rise through the ranks and agrees to this approach ahead of time, unequal partnerships can work just fine.

<u>Equal</u> Partnerships: In these rare partnerships, doctors most often (but not always) have equal shares in the practice and all of it's subsidiaries such as optical shops, buildings, and surgery facilities. Both younger and older doctor partners have an essentially equal voice in management; more decisions are made by consensus rather than formal vote. Perhaps the most important contributor to harmony is that everyone in an equal partnership setting gets an equal share of resources. Marketing dollars are split equally among the various subspecialists. Everyone gets to rotate through the most productive satellite offices. Every doctor gets a turn at the managing partner role. Perhaps most importantly, all partners rise or fall with the total success of the total organization.

Here's an example from a client setting. A large Midwest practice was exploring the admission of a new partner, a well-respected local surgeon who would be merging his smaller solo practice into the larger organization. For the first several hours of our merger conference, the five partners of the larger practice were adamant that the soloist, if he joined, would have to be 100 percent at risk. His compensation methodology was going to be different from everyone else for the first year or two, in a way that we saw was going to potentially result in the new partner's income rising while the old doctor's income fell—or vice-versa.

We suggested that for the first several years the partners might index their split of available profits to their current incomes. If the profits rose 10 percent after the merger, every doctor would get a 10 percent pay raise. All boats would float together. It's interesting to note that as soon as the doctors in the larger group understood the inherent fairness of their incomes rising and falling together based on the success of the entire team, they went on during the rest of our conference to equalize everything else: Access to the best techs, sharing of the evening and weekend hours, and responsibility for covering distant satellite offices.

When two or more doctors draw themselves together, the kind of partnership they choose—equal or unequal—has huge implications for everyone around them. In an equal partnership, the practice administrator is less likely to take sides. In equal partnerships, even junior staff realize that it will be hard to play one doctor off the other. I suspect that even patients get a sense that all doctors are interchangeable, and are more willing to see whichever doctor is most available. I think the reverse is also true. If there's clearly a dominant, "head" doctor, patients gravitate to that one provider, especially for their surgical care. This can amplify rivalries that naturally occur in unequal partnerships.

It's more likely for truly mutual, equal partnerships to form naturally when two young, equally novice doctors start a practice together. Equality is far less common when a young surgeon joins an established doctor 10 years or more ahead in his or her career. In these situations, the young surgeon, even after a successful associateship, will likely remain in the senior doctor's shadow until the older doctor retires, although there can be hope for greater equality with the passage of time. It's been our observation that with age and success, senior ophthalmologists become somewhat less controlling, and more acquiescent to true partner equality. Of course, this usually happens just about the time when the younger generation is wanting to take over and control the practice, themselves, which is why most unequal partnerships stay that way. Perhaps this account will stimulate an internal discussion within your group practice on how authority and control is shared.

A discussion of partnership success models wouldn't be complete without reviewing how young surgeons make it through the ranks from employed associate to partner. We've always been critical of the all or nothing approach most commonly taken in private practice medical employment, where junior doctors are often moved after two or three years, in one great leap, from 'associate' to 'full partner.' This works against basic human nature and the experience of most large institutions (military, educational, religious, trade union, business, political, etc.). These institutions move their members from novice to expert in small, incrementally stages. Perhaps the most intelligent approach to granting partnership in an ophthalmic practice is to grant similar, incremental shares—"merit badges," if you will—so that junior doctors feel a sense of steady progression in their early years.

Whether partners are equal or unequal, the greatest factor for success and harmony is mutual agreement about the development path of the practice. Partnerships are hardest to maintain when there are no large goals held in common—and yet, few group ophthalmology practices have anything like a written business plan. The angriest doctors we counsel are those with partners who don't share their goals, or far worse, hold them back from accomplishing their dreams. In extreme cases, these toxic pairings can lead to the polar opposite of our favorite saying about partners and partnership: "A partner is someone with whom you can accomplish things that you can't accomplish alone."

Finally, some doctors don't really play well in groups, and should probably not be part of a partnership, just as some people should probably not be married. It may take you several years of struggle (or several practice divorces) to learn this about yourself. Fortunately for such doctors, the environment today is allowing eye surgeons who would like to remain solo to do so. With open access to managed care patients, many under-served rural pockets of the country needing doctors, and practice costs that have at least temporarily stabilized as the economy is slowing, solo practice continues to be an option today, and will likely continue to be viable for at least the next generation of surgeons.

There are compelling financial, quality care, lifestyle and existential motivations for a solo surgeon to take on an associate or partner. At the same time, there are compelling and often deeply personal motivations to remain in solo practice. As many larger groups have found, there can actually be severe diseconomies associated with an ophthalmic practice of over three to five partners.

In the years ahead, as the next perplexing rounds of health care cost containment descend on eye care, we believe that many heretofore happy soloists will be at least mildly compelled to consider group practice. The concepts and pearls discussed here, if applied, will help nudge you toward a more profitable enterprise scale, while helping you avoid the most common pitfalls of group practice.

Chapter Fourteen:
ASC Cash Flow Considerations

By Beth Hurley, RN, BSN, CRNO, COE

There are numerous offsetting benefits to taking on the challenges and responsibilities of owning your own ambulatory surgery center (ASC). Most ASC-owning eye surgeons will tell you they wanted more control and the ability to provide efficient, quality surgical care to their patients. Some wanted more convenience in their professional lives. And of course, almost every ASC developer seeks additional revenue to offset falling professional fees.

Developing and managing your own surgical facility present opportunities every week to weigh and balance the numerous trade-offs between cost, quality, outcomes, surgeon preference, and each patient's total experience.

This is true for both the large cost factors—such as facilities, labor, and capital equipment—as well as for the smaller material costs of each case. In the practical, pragmatic era of lower fees that lies ahead, technological sophistication and optimal outcomes must be weighed against cost containment. Each surgeon's wish list must be pared to the resources that deliver the most important patient benefits. None of this is simple for administrators, ASC managers, or medical directors. But it's important to start by defining the mission, goals, and clinical standards of your entire organization, as well as the standards and principles of each constituent surgeon.

Facility Operations

One of the most hotly contested questions in the realm of ophthalmic ASC development is whether a group of surgeons needs one or two operating rooms (ORs). Does it really make sense to run two ORs for a single surgeon operating on a given day? Experience shows that if the facility design is appropriate and the team is well-led, it can be just as time efficient, and significantly less expensive, to run one OR as two.

Several pearls can help you get by with just one room. To run two rooms, you must have two fully equipped and staffed ORs, which can markedly reduce facility profits. A single OR can run just as efficiently—or nearly so—with just a little assistance from the surgeon and anesthesia staff staying actively involved in the turnover process.

If you are developing a new facility or remodeling, be sure to have the sterilization room directly adjacent to the OR so that the next case can be set up while a case is in progress. When the first case is done, the back table is wheeled into the decontamination room by the scrub tech. The surgeon and anesthesia staff take the patient to recovery and get the next patient. The circulating nurse wheels the next case from sterilization into the OR. While the scrub tech uses surgical foam, the circulators reconnect the equipment.

Once the patient is in the room and the surgical site verified, the surgeon foams his or her hands while the surgical tech drapes and anesthesia hooks up monitors. With this kind of choreography and practice, it is quite feasible to transit three or four cases per hour in a single room. Actually, with the simplicity of just one room to worry about, once any routine is defined and everyone knows their role, the team operates more efficiently with fewer errors and less down time for any one staff member.

Even if multiple surgeons presently use your ASC, be sure that utilization is at least 80% on a consistent basis before considering opening a second room—even if nobody wants to operate on Friday afternoons.

As the director of an ASC, you have control over two key expenditure areas: supply costs and staffing costs. Let's review each of these in turn.

The core of ASC materials cost containment is to know your average case cost per surgeon. Before you make any attempts to change, you need to know where you are starting from and obtain current case costs for all your surgeons. For the typical, contemporary cataract surgeon performing topical cases, the average supplies costs inclusive of disposable supplies and IOL now run about $262 per case based on the FASA 2004 ASC Financial Benchmarking Survey, inclusive of the typical $125 paid for the IOL. In thrifty, cost-conscious practices, this can fall to less than $200.

With a baseline understanding of your existing supply costs, you can start a hunt for cost-effective alternatives. Even small savings per case can balloon to major gains in annual ASC profit when multiplied by significant case volumes.

It is easy to become too comfortable with a vendor and its products. On an annual basis, formally review every vendor and every product used. Compare quality, pricing, and service to other alternatives. It's not uncommon to find that when a physician group is wed to the same, single-source vendor for the majority of its surgical supplies, the group pays significantly more than market rates product-by-product.

Look at your facility's sacred cows…things done in the OR because "that's the way it's always been done." Encourage your staff to think out of the box and define why they do it a certain way. For example, I was recently in a facility that used a new bottle of dilating drops for each patient—the contents of the bottle remain sterile unless contaminated by touching the tip of the dropper to any surface—but it had "always been done that way."

Re-evaluate any supplies that are opened but not used. An important cost-savings suggestion is to evaluate what is in the surgical pack on a quarterly basis. Hang an empty bag in the OR and put any supplies that are opened but not used in the bag, even if it is only a pack of spears, a needle, or ten 4 × 4s. The savings add up. It is always more cost efficient to add supplies as needed. (Note that opened and unused supplies can be donated to medical missions.)

Eye surgeons love new equipment and technology. But the overly vanguard adoption of new technology can kill ASC cash flow. Evaluate all new technology with the following in mind:

1. Has it been on the market long enough to reasonably evaluate its cost benefit?
2. Have you talked to other, unbiased users for a recommendation?
3. Will it provide better patient outcomes? How has this been proven? Are the outcomes materially better, or are they a little "iffy"?
4. If patient outcomes will remain the same, will it reduce costs?
5. Will the learning curve be long or short?
6. Will all surgeons at the facility welcome the change, or is there just one proponent for the change?
7. Will it save time—and what is that saved time worth? (For example, consider using a saline lock versus running a TKO IV solution.)

Be thoughtful when you are paying for convenience. A disposable 15 cc bottle of BSS is very convenient and not very expensive, but at an average of $1.25, the savings it may be worth the trouble to fill a reusable bulb. Instead of buying ready-made povidone–iodine 5% solution, mix it 1:1 with BSS and Betadine™ solution 10% at a cost savings of $9.25 per bottle. Anytime you are using a disposable versus a reusable item, it usually costs more for the initial cost. As long as the quality of patient care remains the same, you must then take into consideration the time and cost of preparing or reprocessing.

Know which items are semi-disposable versus being a true one-time-use product. Many manufacturers of surgical blades will provide you with a letter stating that their blade can be re-sterilized, but they will not guarantee the sharpness. With higher case volumes, there can be major savings in using diamond blades versus disposable blades as long as you have a conscientious staff caring for these; repairs are expensive, and a single accident can far outweigh a year of cost savings.

Staffing

Are you using the right person for the right job? With the chronic national nursing shortage, it is time to evaluate what tasks are actually patient care tasks that can only be done by a registered nurse and what tasks can be assigned to a Certified Nursing Assistant (CNA). If you have an RN doing any of the following tasks, it may be time to consider using staff to extend your RNs:

- Walking the patient back to pre-op or out to the car;
- Helping patients to the bathroom or with undressing/dressing;
- Hooking up monitors and taking vital signs;
- Getting patient nourishment; and
- Emptying trash, making beds, turning over rooms, etc.

Remember that Association of periOperative Registered Nurses (AORN) standards require an RN to circulate in the OR and an RN to supervise the pre-op and post-op area.

If there is a nursing school in your area, you may want to consider contacting it to see whether your facility could serve as a training site for clinicals. Although it will not add significantly to your staffing, you will have nurses who are interested in surgery and a chance to have your "pick of the litter" upon graduation.

A typical one-room OR runs most efficiently if cases are scheduled four days a week. A Director of Nurses/Administrator will work five days a week, and the rest of the nursing staff will work four 10-hour days. This would include a total of three RNs—one to circulate in the OR, one in charge of pre-op, and one in charge of post-op—as well as one CNA working between pre-op and post-op and one surgical technician. An additional surgical tech would work five days a week and function as back up to first surgical technician, open cases in the sterilization room, and oversee material management/purchasing. If you are not using an outside janitorial service, a full-time housekeeper can help turn over rooms as well as keep the facility clean throughout the day. In the business office, you would need a business manager who can also do the billing and coding and two front office people who do scheduling, reception, and medical records. In this particular scenario, eight surgeons could use a half day each and readily do 12 cases in four hours.

Remember there are many things outside the surgical schedule that must be done to remain in compliance. Having a day a week without surgical procedures with minimal staff allows time for completion of unpacking and stocking, sterilizing supplies, pulling cases for the next week, and the all-time favorite...PAPERWORK!

Another way to extend staffing is to use office staff. In many facilities, the surgeon's clinical technician can be trained to function as his or her surgical technician. The patients love seeing a familiar face. In addition, clinical staff can be trained to assist in the pre-op and post-op areas, eliminating the need for a CNA.

Purchasing

With the access of Group Purchasing Organization (GPO) services to small ASCs, medical supply distributors have been forced to compete based on their service. A GPO works with manufacturers to obtain better pricing for committed volumes. At no cost, the ASC signs a contract with a GPO to participate and commits to purchasing through that GPO. Once a GPO has been chosen, based on the facilities purchasing needs, the pricing of supplies will be the same regardless of who the medical distributor is. Services to consider when choosing a medical distributor include location of warehouses, on-line ordering, bar coding and scanning, report writing, handling of back orders, extension of payment time up to 60 days, and any additional charges that may apply. With the ability to order and track supplies on-line, it has become much easier to establish, monitor, and contain case costs.

It is important to ensure that your medical distributor will hold at least six weeks of inventory to decrease the effect of back-order situations. This also allows for "just in time" ordering of supplies and will decrease the amount of inventory dollars that are just sitting on the shelf.

Be willing to try new products. Ask your medical distributor to assist you in obtaining samples of items you may want to evaluate for ease of use and cost savings, including sutures, gloves, blades, and any other supplies the facility uses a significant volume of such as IV catheters, syringes, and needles. Encourage the distributor to let you know when a product of comparable quality it available for less cost.

When purchasing equipment, look at alternatives for financing. There are many creative ways when it comes to paying for new equipment such as paying a premium on disposables that allows the facility to pay based on use, 90 days same as cash, and various leasing options. Collaborate closely with your financial advisors for the best long-term cash flow and profit benefits.

Another alternative is to consider used, demo, or remanufactured equipment. Not everything in your equipment inventory has to be bright, shiny, and new. Used stainless steel such as back tables, phaco units, and OR lights are indistinguishable in their function and utility from new equivalents and cost half as much, or less.

Billing and Collections

As covered elsewhere in this chapter, effective patient accounts work requires that you attend to a maddening level of detail and that you never rest in asking new questions. Do you know where your contracts are? When they were last negotiated? Is it better to be contracted or out-of-network? Do you have carve-outs for infrequent/expensive items such as corneal tissue?

Once a contract is negotiated, it is not finished. Contracts should be maintained in a notebook with the date for re-negotiation indicated at the bottom of the binder. Contracts should be reviewed and re-negotiated every year. When payments are received, make sure the payments are correct according to the contract. Request appeals in a timely manner when payments are incorrect.

Many facilities are re-evaluating whether it makes more sense to use out-of-network benefits. Most managed care organizations offer HMO and PPO benefits. If you choose not to contract, you will not be able to provide services to the HMO population, but in most cases you will collect more from the PPO cases. This is important in areas where there is high managed care organization penetration and low reimbursement as a percentage of CMS rates.

Carve-outs are essential if the ASC is doing corneal transplantations or retinal procedures since some of the items used can exceed the total reimbursement for the procedure. In requesting the carve-outs, let the payer know how important it is to provide quality patient care in a cost-effective manner and that it will only be paying for the item if the item is used. Let the payer know you are willing to submit an invoice; be sure to include the cost of shipping and handling.

One way to assess whether you are doing well is to benchmark your accounts receivable with other facilities. These measurements will help recognize areas of performance excellence as well as focus on the areas that have the greatest potential for performance improvement. Both the American Association of Ambulatory Surgery Centers (AAASC) and the Accreditation Association for Ambulatory Health Care (AAAHC) are actively involved in ophthalmic ASC benchmarking studies. When evaluating results, be sure to compare your facility to similar settings.

Regulatory Compliance and Risk Management

I would be remiss to not express here the need to be in compliance with all state and federal regulations regarding the operation of an outpatient surgical facility...as well as the difficulty of doing so. It is of utmost importance that facility managers and owners have the most current resources available. State statutes can be found on-line by contacting the state department of health services. CMS has a website dedicated to ambulatory surgery centers, www.cms.hhs.gov/center/asc.asp. Under the column "Participation" click on "Conditions of Coverage"; then under "Ambulatory Surgical Services" click on "Interpretive Guidelines." This will take you to Appendix L—a document that lists the standards for participation and the interpretive guideline for surveyors.

Other important resource material includes a current copy of "Association of periOperative Registered Nurses (AORN) Standards, Guidelines and Recommended Practices," available on-line at www.aorn.org. Also, access the American Society of Ophthalmic Registered Nurses' (ASORN) (www.asorn.org) "Ophthalmic Procedures: A Nursing Perspective—Operating Room and Ambulatory Surgery Center."

There are many legislative issues, at both the state and federal level, which have a tremendous impact on ASC facility reimbursement. Keep informed with current issues by belonging to and supporting professional organizations such as the American Association of Ambulatory Surgery Centers (AAASC) (www.aaashc.org), the Federal Ambulatory Surgery Association (FASA) (www.fasa.org), and the Outpatient Ophthalmic Surgery Society (OOSS) www.ooss.org. These organizations provide current information regarding changes such as the most current additions and deletions to the ASC list and the status of legislation that ties ASC reimbursement to a percentage HOPS (hospital outpatient services) reimbursement. These organizations all sponsor federal advocacy for ASC issues.

To stay in compliance in an era in which state and Medicare surveys are not consistent, you may want to consider accreditation. Both the Accreditation Association for Ambulatory Health Care (www.aaahc.org) and Joint Commission of Accreditation of Healthcare Organizations (www.jcaho.org) provide accreditation and "deemed status" Medicare surveys. Many states waive state surveys if the ASC facility maintains accreditation. As an additional benefit, accreditation is often looked at with favor—or even required—when contracting with many payer organizations.

Don't forget to protect your assets. Re-evaluate your facility's insurance policies at least every year. Know what (and who) your general liability and business polices cover. It is crucial to understand malpractice insurance coverage as it applies to your facility

Conclusion

For all the myriad details of ASC management and profit enhancement, no single solution works for every facility. Like every segment of your practice enterprise, you must start an ASC with a solid, basic operating foundation from which you can expect very average financial performance and surgical outcomes. After these basics are mastered, additional, incremental gains can be secured. In few other areas of practice management are the twin financial and patient care rewards of making constant small improvements so great as in your own surgery center.

Chapter Fifteen:
Containing Costs and Preserving Practice Liquidity

We hope that some of you are scratching your heads by now and asking, "Hmmm…I thought this was a book on cash flow—isn't the best way to improve cash flow to slash my expenses? Why didn't they talk about cutting costs right up front?" Those excellent questions illuminate a critical flaw in business thinking that is rife in medicine.

Cash flow and profit augmentation in a largely fixed cost service business like eye care is more dependent on revenue enhancement than on cost containment. You simply can't shrink to greatness in this business. Getting cash flowing in the right direction in this business should start first with individual productivity. It's a little bit like riding a bicycle—once you're up to speed, your balance improves and you can think about steering.

All the same, mounds of hard work and positive cash inflow are worthless unless you take steps to taper your expense to a reasonable degree. And it's equally important to develop savings habits that preserve your liquidity during the inevitable ups and downs throughout the year, and to buttress against deeper, but less frequent shocks. Cost containment and liquidity preservation are two sides of the same coin in your practice. Let's cover each of these in turn.

Cost Containment

The most successful cost-containment efforts are spearheaded by one individual who has to drag the rest of the organization along kicking and hollering. But everyone has to get involved to be successful. It works best to push your practice's cost review and cost containment efforts all the way through the organization from the boardroom to the broom closet.

The most difficult challenge is when the office manager or administrator is a lone voice for cost reduction, while the doctors are undisciplined and skip off to the showroom floor to buy their latest whim. As in marriages, practice owners and managers can be on entirely different pages about which costs are essential and which are optional. To the extent possible, be coldly rational, gather the facts about the most profitable course, and let these *facts* make the decision for you.

First and foremost, let reason rule on the gross issue of reasonable profit margins in your practice. We receive calls all the time from doctors concerned that their 35 percent profit margin is unhealthy. Sorry to report, but a 35 percent to 40 percent, profit margin in general ophthalmology (and most subspecialties) is about like a 70-beat heart rate...dead normal. As is a 50-60 percent profit margin in retinal care or a 25-30 percent margin in pediatric eye care. That doesn't mean you can't beat these averages, especially if you have a smaller, solo practice, work in a rural setting, or have a high surgical density practice that comanages. But be realistic. In competitive and expensive urban markets, a 25 percent to 35 percent general ophthalmology profit margin is realistic. If your practice is dominated by capitated HMO patients, a 15 percent profit margin or less is possible.

After looking grossly at your expense and profit margins, we turn to each line item on your income statement. Here are several basic guidelines that you can use as a starting point. Realize, as with all benchmarks, that the most important benchmarking that you do should be to your own historic numbers. You may never be able to get staffing costs down to national averages because of the unique demands of your doctors or patients, but it's real progress to be able to plan for saving, shave a few percentage points off, and then be able to look back and say, "Our profits have gone up 5 percent without a drop in the quality of our care."

Expense Line Item	**Percent Practice Collections**
Auto allowance	0-2 percent
Debt service and lease payments for equipment, working capital, etc.	0-10 percent
Dues, subscriptions, CE/meeting travel	1-2 percent
Equipment warrantees, service, repairs and maintenance	1-2 percent
Facility (total costs including utilities, cleaning and maintenance)	4-6 percent
Insurance (malpractice and general business/liability)	2-5 percent
Local business taxes	0-2 percent
Marketing, advertising and promotion (omitting staff costs)	3-8 percent
Meals and entertainment	1 percent or less
Medical supplies (clinic only)	1 percent or less
Misc: Uniforms, recruiting, licenses, etc.	1+ percent
Office supplies	1-3 percent
Outside billing service (if used, internal staff costs drop)	4-8 percent
Overtime wages at time-and-a-half	1 percent or less
Professional fees (attorney, accountant, consulting, etc.)	2-4 percent
Staff benefits and payroll taxes	3-8 percent
Staff payroll (base wage costs)	15-25 percent
Telephone	1-2 percent

Your practice may be able to get back into alignment by dropping a single expense. For example, an unproductive satellite clinic, or a media advertising contract that just isn't performing. Perhaps a doctor who no longer pulls his own weight needs to go. Don't forget that the fastest way to give owner-doctors a pay raise is to simply terminate an employee doctor and distribute his patients within the remaining group.

What's much more likely, if there are no major costs to contain, will be the need to shave a few dollars from every line item of cost.

Because lay support staffing is the largest expense in most practices, look here first for the greatest opportunities to contain costs. Staffing costs typically consume the first 20 cents to 35 cents of every dollar you collect. But you shouldn't just look at employee costs in the aggregate—you need to assess staffing levels grossly, by department, and by individual contributions and wages. Here's one way to get it done right and fairly to all concerned based on the objective facts.

First, you have to look at the broad practice staffing costs. What percent of your collections go back out for lay staffing, inclusive of wages, taxes and all benefits? For the average general ophthalmology practice in the typical labor market, the target is about 25 percent—lower in successful LASIK or retinal practices, much higher in flagging urban clinics with lower surgical yields. But this is only one gross measure. Another, and perhaps equally valid metric is to divide total annual practice collections by the number of lay staff.

Let's say you have a strong solo practice with $1 million in collections each year. You'll likely have a couple of front desk staff, an office manager or administrator, three or four techs, maybe an outreach or marketing coordinator, and one or one-and-a-half billing staff…let's say nine full-time-equivalents ("FTEs") in all (a full-time-equivalent is a full-time staff member working 40 hours per week.) Do the long-hand division, and that comes to about $111,000 in annual collections per FTE, which is within the normal limits of about $110,000 to $130,000 for the typical well-run practice. Increase staffing just one FTE to 10, and your labor productivity is now $100,000 per FTE-Year; well under normal limits. And if you find a way to get by with 7 FTEs? Your labor productivity climbs to about $143,000 per FTE-Year. But beware! Staffing that's too lean can leave you vulnerable to the loss of just one critical staff member. It's a little like driving your Porsche at the red line for mile after mile. The exhaust whine sounds beautiful, and the ride is thrilling, but when things go wrong, they go wrong catastrophically.

And here's an overlooked option you may not be too conscious of as you're recruiting new staff. Just like the car enthusiast, you need to decide if your practice is going to have a lot of horsepower in reserve and loaf around at 2000 RPM, with everyone loose and easy, or if you're going be running near red line at all times. Most practices err on the side of laxity. We have not evaluated many practices that couldn't lose at least one staff member and sail along just fine the next day. The larger the practice, the greater the odds are that one or two extraneous staff could be terminated without a material impact on operations.

It's a broad generalization, but the most commonly over-staffed area is the techs, and the most often under-staffed area is in patient accounts management. As a result, the most common practice breakdown occurs in billing. Many solo practices are dependent on just one single, key person who is the only staff member who knows how to accurately code, post and submit a charge. If that person goes, the once successful, smaller practice can falter overnight. If you own a small, solo practice and have only one staff member that handles billing work for you, all of the staffing efficiency ideas for you in this article should be overlooked until you have a second backup person who can make sure you get paid for the work you do every month.

Obviously, all of these gross practice ratios break down and look far less favorable if doctors don't' do their parts. If you're the owner of a $1 million practice, and generate $180 per average patient visit, you're likely to have labor statistics that are far more favorable than if you generate just $125 per patient visit. In the latter case, it will take more tech time, more patient accounts work, and more marketing oomph, simply because you'll have to drive 44 percent more patients in the front door to generate the same cash flow. Your staffing costs probably won't be 44 percent higher, but profitability and staffing efficiency will be lots worse off. *And*, don't forget that you'll personally have to work 44 percent harder. So part of the staffing efficiency challenge is to increase your <u>personal</u> productivity, including the procedural and special testing density of your practice.

Let's next examine your practice's staffing efficiency by department, starting with the most expensive segment, technical staffing. Every eye surgeon has their own preferences for how they use lay staff to support patient care. And most approaches work just fine in an environment with sufficiently high fees. We know surgeons who can transit 80 or more patients a day with two technicians, and other surgeons who could not get through 35 patients without 5 techs in attendance. In the former case, that's just 0.2 tech payroll hours per patient visit. In the latter case, 1.1 tech payroll hour per visit. The normal metric, averaged over a year for a general ophthalmology practice, should be 0.6 to 0.8 tech payroll hours per patient visit. For a high-volume surgical practice, with lots of short, postoperative visits, you should be able to hit the lower end of this range. For a testing intensive retinal practice, the tech labor number will typically be somewhat higher (0.9+ tech payroll hours pet patient visit), but then, so too will the economic yield of each patient. What should shine through this discussion is that any nationally published norms—including what you are reading here—should be secondary to your own sense of the internal benchmarks in your unique practice. You should measure these norms, and then work hard to beat your own numbers, <u>especially</u> if your figures fall outside of national averages.

What doesn't work very well or efficiently is for your eye clinic to use highly paid technicians as glorified runners or to use optometrists instead of technicians to work up patients. For that matter, it isn't wise to work patients up yourself and "double-pass" them, seeing patients twice during a single visit, both before and after they have been dilated.

Next, we turn to the patient accounts department. If yours is the typical general practice with the typical mix of services and payers, and everyone does their part at the front desk and in the clinic to accurately enter each patient's demographics and to correctly code diagnoses and services, you should be able to get by with one patient account staffer for every $800,000 to $1.2 million in annual collections, as we have covered elsewhere in this book. But different circumstances dictate different numbers. Let's say you practice in Southern California or Southern Florida or in selected rust-belt cities. These are places where higher managed care penetration gives you a triple whammy of upping the need for pre-authorization, reducing payments and adding considerable time and bureaucratic friction in claims submission and processing. The best you may be able to do in such settings is $600,000 in annual collections per patient accounts staffer per year.

As you can see from the discussion so far, the most favored practices are in rural parts of the country—labor costs (as well as facility and most other costs) are low, managed care penetration is low, and the revenue per patient visit can be high, because there is little competition and more surgery to go around. As a result, practice profits in well-run rural organizations are 50 percent or higher, and you can afford to be a little looser with staffing efficiency. If you only spend 17 percent on staffing, who really cares if you have an extra runner on the clinic floor to do personal errands for the doctors? At the opposite extreme, urban, managed care havens may be exciting markets to live in (Manhattan, San Francisco, Boca Raton) but they are horrendous markets in which to contain staffing costs. The most enticing markets to live in are populated with eye surgeons making 25 percent profit margins in the best years. In point of fact, the happiest eye surgeons we've ever met with on the Upper East Side were doctors there on vacation from places like Arkansas, Oklahoma and North Dakota.

It's hard to measure reception and check-out staff productivity without a close study of their functions in your practice. But for the typical job description, including checking patients in and out, screening phone calls for the entire office, short-stopping prescription refills and pre-op instruction confusions, scheduling and re-scheduling patients, making new appointments, and taking the heat from all sides, you can expect one receptionist or checkout clerk for about every 400 patients per month, give or take a hundred patients. Nowhere are small differences in productivity more apparent—we've seen 1,000+ patients per month practices handled by solo front desk super stars, and fragile, under-trained clerks flummoxed by a quarter of this volume. Tenure, maturity, work-hardening and solid skills make all the difference in the world. When you finally get the right person in place, give them money and prizes to make them stay. They are the overlooked key to practice success, and the beating heart of the most outstanding practices in America.

What about optical productivity? Look for something in the range of $150,000 to $225,000 in annual optical sales per full time equivalent, or recast in other terms, spending about 25 percent to 33 percent of optical sales on staffing for this department. There are a lot of "it depends" in this area, too. If you sell a strong line of premium goods, or push the edge on mark-ups, the percentile staffing costs should be lower. If you run your optical purely as a patient convenience (and you shouldn't), with lower markups, expect staffing costs to be higher as a percent of total sales.

For practices large enough to have a formal marketing department, this is probably one of the least accountable areas of labor productivity, though this need not be the case. Depending on what kind of marketing you engage in, your marketing staff could potentially be the most accountable part of your team, especially if you focus first efforts (as you should) on the interior of the practice: Recall, patient satisfaction, alumni referral development and real service to your referring doctors. Each of these areas are exquisitely subject to results measurement. Not so, of course, general consumer advertising, where the return-on-investment gets fuzzy, fast. Bottom line? It's reasonable for the average practice for marketing (inclusive of relevant staffing costs) to cost 3-8 percent of each dollar collected. The most common mistake made is for clients to sink substantial sums into external marketing before they have fully drilled into the un-tapped internal pools of patients through recall and alumni referral development.

How about that department of one—the office manager or administrator of your practice? With rare exception, this person is the most competent member of the staff, yet they don't often enjoy the full confidence of doctor-owners. As a result, too much of their time is taken up in validating their worth to the boss, and too little time is spent doing what the best managers do best: increasing the productivity and morale of every other worker—lay and doctor—in the company.

Of course we need to insert a little heresy here for at least half of our readers: *It's not absolutely essential that you have an administrator or office manager.* In fact, we've seen practices ranging to $4 million in annual collections with strong department heads, very engaged doctors, a few consultants on call, and no administrator. They seem to survive for years on end just fine. It's not the best approach in most settings, because few doctors have the patience to lead their lay team, but demonstrates that anything is possible if required by the circumstances. Most practices without an administrator don't plan to run like that, but are just driven to this model because they can't find or keep a competent individual on board.

Now let's turn to the matter of individual staff productivity vs. their compensation. The former, productivity, should be judged by individual department managers. Semi-annual staff evaluations should include a rating for raw production, even if this has to be subjective and judgmental, as may be the case for front desk staff. Most other areas of the practice can be finitely measured. As an example, assign a different highlighter pen to every tech, and have them mark the patient schedule posted at the nurses station—you can easily count each tech's daily workups and reach useful conclusions about individual productivity.

Individual compensation for each position in the practice should be reviewed annually against local standards. If you want to have a small, crack staff of "commandos," it may make sense to pay a small team in the upper range of local standards. This may be appropriate for higher-demand/higher-profit surgical referral center practices. If, by contrast, your practice has a high percentage of low-profit-margin, routine eye care patients, it may be more appropriate to employ a larger team with less skill and lower pay, just to mush the needed raw numbers through the organization.

Here's the final examination of your practice's staffing costs. If you have a general practice, don't work in a managed care hot bed, don't have unusually stiff competition, and don't have eccentric doctors with extreme support demands, you should fit within the following norms:

- Annual revenue per lay FTE per year: $110,000 to $130,000;
- 20 percent to 33 percent of collections spent on lay staff wages, taxes and benefits;
- 0.6 to 0.9 tech payroll hours per patient visit, averaged over the year;
- An "office manager" earning $45,000 and up for practices with $1 million in annual collections; or an "administrator" earning another $10,000 or so above this for about every extra half-million in annual collections per year up to a peak salary of roughly $200,000 per year in the largest practices. Alternately, you can potentially forego an administrator if you have an engaged managing partner and a strong team of middle managers;
- Optical sales of at least $200,000 per dispensing optician;
- An executive assistant, shared by the administrator and doctors, once annual collections reach $2 million or more;
- In-house marketing support to the extent that total marketing costs, inclusive of payroll, don't exceed 8 percent for a mature general practice or 15 percent for a mature and established refractive surgery practice (practices growing and consciously increasing investments in marketing can reasonably spend at twice these levels and still be rational);
- A full-charge in-house bookkeeper, part- or full-time, once annual collections reach $3 million or more; and
- A full-time human resources director once your headcount exceeds about 100 FTEs.

If your practice is off in one or more areas, consider staffing up or down to fall within norms. At the very least, visit a colleague's practice that falls within normal limits to see how they get by, or furlough one or more staff to see how a busy day can really get by just fine within the extra assistance. For strong practices, right-sizing will make a material difference in profitability with the continued fee cuts. For already-weak practices, getting to the right number of support staff will be necessary for survival over the balance of this challenging decade.

Now let's wrap our minds around spending in some of the other major areas of the practice. Promotional expenses are the number two or number three cost in practices. We've already covered marketing cost containment in Chapter Eleven. So next we move to facility costs.

Facility cost analysis breaks into several logical areas. Most broadly, should you lease your facility or own your own office? Many dependent variables plug into this important question:

1. How important is owning your own building to you? This is a book about cash flow, but the number one driver for putting up your own facility is often not money but ego. If it would please you to drive up to your own facility, this pleasure may reasonably trump minor cost or cash flow issues. After all, you and your staff spend more waking hours each week in your office than anywhere else. Why shouldn't it be a pleasurable, prideful, chest-swelling experience?

2. How available is rental space in your market? How available are appropriate land parcels or buildings to buy? You may be constrained in one direction or another by the answers.

3. How dependent are you on referrals from a hospital campus? Let's say you're shoehorned into cramped space on campus now, paying outrageous rent. Your first thought might be to move off campus and establish a freestanding office. Think again, if an appreciable percentage of your new patients come from doctors on campus, who might take poorly to your appearance of defection.

4. How stable and predictable is your growth? If your practice is growing rapidly, or it's trajectory is unpredictable, it may be better to lease for a few years, rather than rent.

5. How volatile is your practice? A doctor with ups and downs should probably not be locked into owning a fixed-size building or even into signing a long-term lease. Instead, wait for stability, or at the very least, commit to the smallest possible space.

6. How organized are you? If you are already having a hard time managing a medical practice, would you be able to organize a building project?
7. What promotional benefit would you get from your own freestanding space? Most doctors get a major lift in their revenue when they move to a new office that they've just built. Frankly, we're unable to say whether this is because they feel renewed pressure to produce, or they really attract more customers.
8. Where do you and your advisors believe local property values will head in the future? This is a major determinant and difficult to assess at present. Some thoughtful experts feel we're in a property valuation bubble, and that prices will pop shortly; other, equally thoughtful pros feel real estate will continue to be a great investment. Making this more complex is that specialized medical space for an ophthalmic office has a much smaller market of potential buyers, and those buyers will be under increasing pressure to contain costs over the next 10-30 years—the window in which you will likely sell your building.
9. Where do you believe interest rates are heading? As this book goes to press, we are at historically low mortgage interest rates. This should drive you a little closer to a "build" or "buy" rather than "lease" decision, but of course, property values are also at an all-time high.
10. What's your succession plan? Owning your (solo) practice building can sometimes make transfer of your practice to the next doctor-owner more difficult by increasing the overall price of the transaction, unless you elect to keep the building and lease it back to the new practice owner. In group practices, adding the cost of buying into the building as well as the practice may reduce the price partner-track associates are willing to pay for other elements of the practice's value, such as goodwill.

Bottom line? Near and intermediate term, it can cost more—even a lot more—to own your office facility. But longer-term, it almost always pays to be an owner. If, instead of paying 4-6 percent of your collections on rent and utilities, you can afford in cash flow terms a few years of paying 8-12 percent, and grow into your facility costs as your practice grows, then you should take the plunge.

Now, how about those dozens of other line items of expenditure in the practice besides the Big Three, staffing, facilities, and marketing? Unfortunately, as an administrator or doctor, you may not be very aware of the spending details way down in the trenches. Is too much inventory kept on hand? Are vendors chosen for personality rather than price and service? Do the doctors need to converge their brand preferences so a better volume discount can be negotiated with one preferred vendor?

To help with this, hold department-by-department meetings with staff and poll them for cost-saving ideas. You may want to consider a financial incentive for such staff ideas (e.g.: $50 paid each month for the best cost-containment suggestion.) Ultimately, someone in the company at a senior level has to be aware of the details of every line item of expense. An owner should be signing all checks above an agreed amount (with invoices always attached and the bookkeeper or administrator on hand to answer questions), and the same doctor or a different doctor should be reviewing the monthly general ledger.

For the average practice, with a competent administrator, all expenses below $500 can be OK'd by the administrator. Expenses (except for pre-approved standing costs in the budget) that exceed $500 should be approved by the managing partner or another designated owner. MUCH higher amounts, such as approving a new staff position or a new piece of $20,000 capital equipment, should be approved by the board or the executive committee. In tight circumstances, it may be appropriate to decrease every manager's and doctor's spending authority, or to install a more formal purchase order system. In larger practices, it can pay to centralize the purchasing, stocking and inventorying function to a single agent.

Here's another dimension of cost and cash flow containment: Examine your payables aging, and stretch this out to every possible, ethical extent. Remember that we're trying to enhance profits; it's not going to be helpful if in stringing out a vendor you stimulate retaliatory pricing or incur late fees. In today's world, it's overly-generous to pay upon receipt of an invoice. In most circumstances, a 30-day float will be well accepted, and you may be surprised to find that a much longer payment cycle is yours for the asking. Also, don't pass up the common 2 percent savings that some vendors grant for early payment.

Many of your practice's vendors, especially if we enter any periods of deflation in the years ahead, may be even more generous. In the words of one corporate trainer who specializes in negotiating skills, "You don't get what you deserve you get what you negotiate." Let's examine how this sentiment applies more than ever to your practice today. It may be possible to negotiate your way to at least slightly higher profits.

In other business sectors, where normal profit margins can be 10 percent or less, shaving even a point or two from the raw costs of delivering a product or service boosts profits hugely. If you were a restaurateur or electronics manufacturer, wringing out small vendor and labor concessions could make the difference between failure and success.

In the first wave of cost cutting that swept through practices more than a decade ago, managers and owners gave up the marginal items they could do without...things like patient transport or post-op gifts. They also started to cut away those things they could do for themselves in-house, like monthly accounting tasks, made easier with the new generation of accounting packages. They started asking staff to pay for soda in the break room. If you are reaching limits on what you can eliminate categorically, it may be time to delve back into each line item of non-removable expense to see how you can cut costs within each category. The results of this refined cost containment won't buy a Lear jet, but it could help to keep you flying level during the next few rounds of fee reductions.

Rather than focusing on one or two areas of the practice, examine every category for even modest reductions. In aggregate, small pricing concessions for products or services you use regularly over many years will add up enormous bottom-line yields. And even if a vendor has no room to move price-wise, they may be able to add value to the overall exchange that saves costs in other dimensions—for example a computer vendor who can be coaxed into enriching your contract with free training sessions or an extended warrantee period.

The typical practice writes about 200 checks a month to a wide range of vendors. Over the course of a year, there may have been 500 different parties who sold you their services or products.

You may believe that some of these vendors have a steel claw on your practice purse, but even statutory expenses may not be mandatory. One of your obliged vendors is the postal service. Now you can't negotiate down the price of a first-class stamp, but you can certainly get a bulk rate postal permit. Spring should be open hunting season on virtually every vendor relationship your business maintains.

Here's an easy exercise. Assemble the practice's most senior staff. Get out your checkbook or general ledger. For every vendor (including some of the less obvious ones, like Sally at the front desk) fill out the following simple form:

Vendor Name	Cost Per Year	Current Rating (Superior, Acceptable, Probationary or Terminable)	Our Ability to Eliminate or Substitute	Agreed Action
Mike's Office Cleaning Service	*$6000*	*Superior—always exceed our expectations, and no rate increase in 5 years*	*Lot's of options, but no need to replace.*	*Letter of thanks for another great year of service.*
First Federal Bank & Loan	*$800*	*Terminable—refused to increase our credit line, and lots of statement errors*	*Three other banks available within one mile; all have agreed to waive account fees.*	*Interview branch managers and change banks by July 1st.*
Amy Young, Junior Tech	*$34000*	*Probationary—after 18 months on the floor, she's still not able to refract; in addition, although she is pleasant to patients she continues to have mild conflicts with her supervisor.*	*Techs are hard to find in our market, but during the summer slow season we can do with one less tech*	*Provide Amy with one last written warning and 6 weeks to shape up between now and July 15; terminate PRN and replace by September 1st.*
McLauren Advertising	*$225000*	*Acceptable—This vendor is sufficient for our immediate needs, but may not have the creativity if we expand our LASIK program.*	*The best ad agency in town already serves our competitor; we've gotten too big for most freelancers; the next step may be to create an in-house department.*	*Meet with our account executive and tell them we're expecting more this year, or we will commence a formal agency review in the 4th quarter; review bills closely.*

Here are some cost-containment or service enhancement opportunities you may have overlooked:

- Ask companies with a discount policy for prompt payment (eg: 2 percent off for payment within 10 days) to extend that same discount if you pay at the 30-day mark;

- Ask your cleaning service what discount they would provide if you had each staff member take a moment to bag their own paper waste at the end of the day, or if they cleaned the office just three times a week instead of five times during the slow winter months;

- Ask ongoing, reliable vendors (eg: radio stations you advertise on and similar small, flexible businesses) if they can provide you with an additional discount for a longer-term contract, or for pre-paying for a year of service. If your practice has sufficient cash or borrowing power, at current interest rates, a 10-15 percent discount for pre-payment may be strongly in your favor;

- Ask the wall paper hanger what discount they could provide on the total job if they not only papered the office, but the homes of five staff members and doctors who have been wanting to redecorate their residences;
- Ask your optical frame vendors what further discount you would enjoy if you bought just four frame lines instead of the current 12, and could push more business to a smaller number of companies;
- Ask your techs if some of them would be willing to job-share and take 15 hours of work off each week during the slowest times of the year;
- Ask your optometrist if he/she would be willing to see just four more patients a day, which would conservatively generate another $100,000 in annual revenue;
- Ask your staff if they would be willing to launder their own uniforms, saving $3,500 in cleaning service fees each year;
- Ask you patients if they would be willing to use the office's courtesy telephone to call their own insurance company for approvals, or to call for a taxi cab at the end of an appointment, thus saving the practice valuable staff time;
- Ask the director of the open access LASIK center you use if you can perform your low number of cases at their "high volume discount rate" for the next 12 months while you build your practice;
- The next time you need an exam room full of equipment, ask your equipment vendor to bid it out both ways, new and refurbished/used;
- If you use a hospital's outpatient department to perform cataract surgery, ask the PR department to help you with a publicity project for free, saving you the cost of hiring a local freelance publicist;
- If you haven't checked your carrier's long-distance phone rates against the competition in the last year, check them now—they're falling like a rock. At the very least, ask your current carrier if they have a less-costly plan for a customer like you;

- Ask the sandwich shop that caters your staff lunch every week if they can throw in dessert for free since you're such a great customer;

- Ask your local postmaster if there's a less costly (or less time-consuming) way you could mail out patient statements;

- Ask your doctors if they could be a little less wordy in their dictation to save transcription costs;

- Ask yourself if you really need to send eight staff members across the country to a meeting, or could the same training goal be accomplished by sending the most deserving two staff members, and having them be the in-house trainers for the other six;

- Ask yourself if a $59 accounting software package and three extra hours a month of your office manager's time could eliminate most of the $6,000 annual bill you get from your accountant....and get you more timely financial reports in the bargain; and

- Ask if annual dues paid to umpteen local, state and national professional societies, along with licensure renewals in multiple states, is still necessary at this point in your life, or do you no longer have a need to pad your CV?

The purpose of this annual exercise is not to dump your vendors. Indeed, it may remind you to praise both internal and external vendors who are truly superior. Depending on the vendor, the action you take may include asking for better pricing, better payment terms, or better services. Make this pruning and weeding process an annual habit, an annual rite of spring, and your practice garden will bloom better in each successive year.

Enhancing Practice Liquidity

Novelist W. Somerset Maugham once wrote: "Money is like a sixth sense, without which you cannot make a complete use of the other five." Most ophthalmologists are reminded of this in the first few months of every year. The first-quarter profits in the majority of practices tumble with a slew of seasonal adversities.

With the onset of winter, and the departure of snowbirds from northern latitudes, about half of the country's eye surgeons have a drop in elderly patient volume. (Of course, this is offset in southern practices, where the snowbirds roost.) What's more, snow days can slaughter an entire week of patients in the toughest climates.

Physician vacation time is also often at a peak in the winter, not only for legal holidays, but for vacations south (for some) and to the ski slopes (for the rest.)

The start of every New Year can predictably take certain expenses up a notch, and certain payments to the practice down a notch. Taken together, it's no wonder that we get a large percentage of our calls for help at the start of the year. There are year-end lease escalations, cost of living raises for staff, increased utility costs and annual vendor price hikes. At the same time, physician draws from the practice increase to catch up with any under-funded tax deposits and to cover holiday vacation spending.

Medicare payments slow down as patients try to delay as long as possible the cost of the New Year's deductible. Optical sales are sluggish, as the buying public shakes off their holiday spending hangovers.

None of these individual hits are all that traumatic. But taken together, they can shove weak practices over the cliff and nudge even the strongest practices into a short-term deficit. In the last decade, these oscillations into first quarter deficits have been getting just a little worse each year. This normal, seasonal tumble has been exaggerated in the most recent years in refractive surgery practices, which are weathering a continued recession in most parts of the country (and slowly coming back elsewhere, as new technology is being introduced.)

It's now a perfect time to discuss how you can get off the unpleasant roller coaster, or at least smooth out your ride by the time the *next* winter lull arrives. Let's review four simple lessons.

Lesson Number One: The Practice Treasury

All countries have a treasury department, and many keep significant reserves—real treasure, as in gold bars, or at least their infinite taxing authority, backed by military power—to back their currency and as a store of national wealth. Most corporations of any stature also follow a strict treasury protocol, keeping a portion of their capital locked up as a reserve against future calamity and future opportunity. In a roundabout fashion, mature eye surgery practices have a kind of "treasury"—it's not gold bars kept in a vault, but the personal wealth of the constituent surgeons. If the practice hits a lull, the doctors can simply forego their salaries for a few months. If the lull is prolonged, the owners can make a loan to the practice.

Younger doctors and surgeons that are less careful with their personal wealth often don't have this cushion. They can't forego a salary, and they can't make a loan to their practices. We've consulted with several such surgeons recently, surgeons hit with the quintuple whammy of a recession, September 11, a portfolio of depressed tech stocks, and an excess focus on LASIK surgery, all on top of the usual first-quarter blahs. Many of these doctors now face corporate or personal bankruptcy because they didn't have sufficient reserves on hand.

How much in reserves is enough? This is a complex question, with several interconnecting parts. How fast is the practice growing and what are your profit margins? If profit margins are low, you have less cushion for error or a general economic slide, than if your margins are high. What about your lifestyle costs? If you have painted yourself into the corner with an unalterable $500,000 annual lifestyle, and the practice generates $520,000 a year, things will get rough with just one more Medicare fee cut. Remember that a man who makes just a dollar a day is rich if he can live on 50 cents.

How old are you? If you are 40, and have 25 years to recover from a business miscalculation, you don't need the reserves of a 60-year-old. How large and how vulnerable is your retirement portfolio? If you're nearing retirement age, and financially secure, there's nothing wrong with taking one last, dicey, business fling, or coming close to burning up your practice's reserve cash.

Lesson Number Two: Working Capital Loans and Credit Lines

Some practices are more cyclical than others. This is largely related to practice location and the "snowbird-effect." If you don't have a reserve account, a "treasury," built up yet to buffer the highs and lows of the practice, you critically need to arrange credit facilities. One or more lines of credit are important to negotiate and have in place, at the ready, before you need them. Again, it's reasonable to have three to six months of practice overhead at your ready disposal.

Lesson Number Three: Disability and Life Insurance

Entire books could be devoted to discussing the appropriate disability and life insurance coverage for surgeons in various circumstances. For the sake of brevity, simply understand that the chief difficulty of planning for personal disaster is imagining that disaster can happen in the first place. Seek out one or more competent local advisors (your accountant, fee-only planner or insurance broker) and take their advice on the proper level of coverage to meet your circumstances. With any proposed policies in hand from your friendly insurance broker, be sure to validate that you are striking an appropriate balance between being under- and over-insured, and that the right products are being employed, by talking to your accountant before signing.

Lesson Number Four: Annual Budgets

Underlying this chapter's discussion is the concept that you need to be able to forecast various contingent scenarios, and then play though all of the "what ifs?" The ideal starting point is to have an annual budget for your practice. If you can lay out the month-by-month expected revenue and expenses, it's much easier to do contingency planning. With Excel or any similar spreadsheet program, you can quickly assess the impact of losing a doctor from a practice, closing down a satellite office or dropping out of a managed care plan. This budget should be prepared in the last quarter of every year, and be laid side-by-side with your monthly and year-to-date financial statements. Some doctors and managers complain that drawing up a budget in advance is too constraining. On the contrary, having a budget will give you new freedoms to explore options that before you were not precisely sure were possible. The only thing that a proper budget might constrain is your odds of going out of business.

Economic risk management and contingency planning is not yet a common, *formal* management discipline in ophthalmic circles, even though it's going on all the time intuitively and informally. It's fascinating to note that one of the truly excellent texts of practice financial management, Financial Management for Medical Groups, by Earnest Pavlock (published by the Medical Group Management Association) still has no index citations for either the word "liquidity" or the word "reserves." This would be unheard of in a general business finance and accounting text, but not entirely surprising, since the typical medical practice runs double-digit profit margins, while the typical "real" business more often runs single-digit profits, or at best profits in the low teens. As the operating margins of ophthalmology realistically come to ever more resemble the margins in general business, we'll all have to master the language, the habits *and the caution* of our colleagues in these more commercial environments.

Chapter Sixteen: A Tale of Two Oregon Practices... Cash Flow Difficulties, Opportunities, and Lessons Learned

By Laurie K. Brown, COMT, COE
Belinda Baldwin, CPC
Drs. Fine, Hoffman & Packer, LLC, Eugene, Oregon

Elizabeth Cottle, CPC
Casey Eye Institute, Portland, Oregon

[Editors Note: We have combined what were originally planned for two separate guest chapters in this book into a single chapter to contrast several issues. First and foremost to show how the concepts in this text translate into practical use in the field. Second, to illustrate useful operational details. And third, to hold up in sharp contrast the implementation hurdles in larger institutional settings as compared to smaller private practices. The pace at which you are able to implement the concepts in this book will be bounded only by the scale of your organization and your zeal to reform. It's clear that all improvements in practice cash flow and patient accounts management are best accomplished through constant small improvements rather than sweeping change.]

From Drs. Fine, Hoffman & Packer, LLC, Eugene, Oregon

Protocols are key in medical practice cash flow management. Our Financial Policy is what we use to communicate our expectations regarding patients' financial responsibility. Our Collection Policy is the protocol our practice follows to ensure we are being paid efficiently for the services we provide to our patients. These policies help us to make certain that our accounts receivable are collected in a timely manner and that our guidelines are applied consistently to all patients. Both protocols start with patient and staff education.

Patient education must begin at the first encounter with the practice, prior to their visit. We obtain preliminary insurance information from our patients when scheduling their appointment. Our new patient packet, sent in advance of the patient's first appointment, includes a welcome letter, practice brochure (including a paragraph summarizing our Financial Policy), insurance information sheet (which details managed care and referral processes), and our Financial Policy. Upon check-in for their first visit, new patients are given another a copy of our Financial Policy and asked to provide their signature attesting to their understanding of the policy. This form is kept in the patient chart.

Staff education is necessary to empower each employee to confidently educate our patients regarding our policies and collect dollars owed for services rendered. Our Collection Policy helps to build employee confidence and understanding, eliminating self-doubt, and empowering our staff to comfortably ask for payment from our patients. An employee who is unsure of exactly what fees are due will hesitate and put off asking patients for payment of their co-pays, account balances and their portion of current charges for which they are responsible.

All front office staff have quick reference sheets at their fingertips which remind them of how to ask for payments and give them problem solving phrases to help them give patients suggestions to overcome obstacles in making payments. We strive to keep our overhead expenses to a minimum whenever possible and it certainly helps to not have to send out statements for balances that could have been easily collected at the time of service.

Collections start with our initial contact with patients and continue throughout our entire relationship. Our computer system has a feature that will make a collection message flash on a patient's account screen. When making the patient's next appointment, the flashing message is a sign to the scheduler to identify that the patient's collection status is delinquent. This gives our staff the opportunity to remind the patient of any outstanding balance prior to their next visit. Any additional billing information needed, such as an updated address, "flashes" for the scheduler as well.

A few days prior to the patient's visit, we check for appropriate referrals and highlight any outstanding balances on the patient's superbill or fee slip for the next visit. If a staff member has a question about a patient's collection status, they can then communicate with the office manager in advance of a patient's appointment. Delinquent accounts that have been turned over to a collection agency in the past are considered "self-pay" accounts unless insurance benefits have been verified prior to the visit.

Our check-in receptionist verifies insurance and personal demographic information when greeting the patient. This is also the time to collect any insurance co-pays for the day's visit. Our check-out receptionist acts as a back-up for collecting co-pays and any outstanding personal balances from prior visits, in addition to collecting deductibles, non-covered services (such as refractions from Medicare patients), and total visit charges for uninsured patients as they leave our office. If patients state that they are unable to pay their bills at the time of service, the check-out receptionist will re-educate them about our policy so they can be prepared at their next visits. In addition, these patients are given self-addressed envelopes so they can mail in their balance for the day's charges. (This is another way to reduce costs by not having to send unnecessary statements.)

We post our charges to patient accounts on the same day for morning appointments and the next day for afternoon appointments. The information comes from the superbill where the physician has recorded the CPT and ICD-9 codes. At the end of each day we account for all superbills by preparing a reconciliation report. All fee slips are reviewed for possible charges missed and co-pay collection as part of the end-of-day process. If a co-pay was not collected at the time of service, a "co-pay form letter" is sent to the patient with a self-addressed envelope for their use.

We review all paper claims for insurance ID, referral numbers, modifier need, and any other appropriate information that may be missing, prior to being sent. We want to ensure that our claims are accurate to reduce denials and get paid in a timely manner. All Medicare and other electronic claims are sent out daily. Our computer system has a feature that will "kick out" electronic claims if there is information missing.

Our collection policy details that statements should be run daily as part of the end-of-day process. Patients receive a statement every 30 days. We bring the patients' attention to balances owed for greater than 30 days by a bright green "overdue" sticker. For balances over 60 days, a bright red "10 day final notice" is placed on the patients' statement. We then follow up with a phone call in 10 days if the balance remains outstanding. We make an effort to collect the balance via credit card when we have the patient on the phone. If a payment has not been made, and the patient does not attempt to make payment arrangements after a third 90 day statement is sent, then the balance will be sent to a collection agency. (If the debt is under ten dollars it will be written off as a "bad debt" and the account flagged with a flashing collection message for the next visit.)

We produce a "pending insurance" report every other week to allow us to check on any claims outstanding greater than 45 days. We will then either re-file the claim with a "second request" note, or call the insurance company to check on the claim status. A monthly accounts receivable report is prepared, and we aim for a high collection standard in each of these three categories: Insurance, personal, and combined balances. We aim for 60 percent of accounts within 30 day, 20 percent in 30-60 day, 10 percent in 60-90 day, 5 percent in 90-120 day, and 5 percent in the greater than 120-day categories. Our practice has learned that persistence and tireless attention to all the cash flow details discussed here give us security in the health of our business and in all of our futures, which depend on the practice success.

We review our fee schedule annually with careful calculations to ensure that our fees are appropriate for our area and specialty. This is also the time when we open the "wish list" file of superbill/fee slip procedure and diagnostic code changes so that the superbill can be updated to reflect our most current utilization needs and ideas for increased efficiency. We develop those ideas over the preceding year for use in this very important tool.

Practice protocols of all types require employee cooperation and knowledge. Training and cooperative work are accomplished by keeping staff familiar with the protocols. This is done by periodic but routine reviews, especially at times when changes are made and implemented. We strive to maintain a caring attitude throughout our entire relationship with our patients. Every staff member must realize the importance of working together as a team and their individual part in the collection process. The patient is a part of our team and deserves to be educated to our expectations, fairness and consistency. The Golden Rule applies here as it does with everything we do; treating others as we want to be treated is our best policy.

From the Casey Eye Institute, Portland, Oregon

The Casey Eye Institute in Portland, Oregon is a large university department of ophthalmology for Oregon Health & Science University. The six-floor facility has its own surgical suites specializing in ophthalmic surgery, and represents every subspecialty in the field. There are twenty-eight ophthalmologists, four optometrists, four ophthalmic fellows and twelve residents. Besides providing outpatient hospital care and surgery, the faculty has a private practice whose billing is provided by an outside service.

We were faced with a number of challenges. The size and scope of practice has provided many operational challenges and opportunities for improvement. Due to the design of the building and the fact that each sub-specialty has its own reception area, patients have many points of entry into the system. There are a total of eleven locations, including two retail-type services for optical and contact lenses. The opportunity for transactions (and mix-ups) was further increased by the variety of staff included in each of these areas. Front desk staff collect co-pays, the cosmetic and refractive centers collect up front for surgery and non-insured patients may also be asked for a deposit on a planned surgery.

No cash drawers or cashier staff had been established, thus we were an "exact change only, please" practice, and also accept personal checks and Visa/MasterCard. Staff had been inconsistent in their requests for co-pays to be paid at the time of service. Since we use an offsite billing service, cash was being sent via courier in a locking bank bag. However, staff performed no reconciliation against the schedule versus co-pays requested/received or the receipt book, versus what was sent to billing office and what arrived in billing office. Plus, the existing process did little to reduce the potential for theft.

The project ahead of us was formed through a task force team. Department administration hired an outside accountant for an audit of the existing process and to make recommendations. This was decided for 'buy-in' impact on faculty and staff, rather than recommendations coming from an internal staff person. Through our department's Performance Improvement Committee, a separate task force was formed to analyze the issues, design a workable policy and implement the plan via training. The team consisted of representatives from the billing office, one of the retail shops, the accounting department and a front desk person.

We came up with the following plan...

- Improve consistency of co-pay collection via our scheduling system, which is able to provide prompts on the daily printed schedule.
- Create scripts to aid staff on how to ask for payment.
- Assign a staff member to act as a cashier on each of the two main clinical floors, with a trained substitute. The cashier would be available to make change only. The responsibility for obtaining a co-pay and turning in the money remains with division staff.
- Assign the cashier the following duties: Count, balance, and log the cash drawer daily. We took a short step back by creating a pegboard receipt book, which provides the patient with their receipt and logs the entry at one time. The log can then be totaled for the day and submitted. The log is then counter-signed by a supervisor.

- Place cash collected in a lock box at end of each day, with the log-sheet and a copy of the schedule showing amounts expected and collected.
- Assign accounting staff to retrieve cash from the lock box, verify amounts received from divisions, with batch cash going to billing office with a grand total.
- Require the billing office to verify the correct amount was received by having a staff member sign the batch form and return it to the accounting office.
- Monitor the new process with occasional mystery shoppers and random audits of records.

Based on our early experience with this new process, employee consistency in asking for money has improved. Altering existing staff duties to add cashiering has proven difficult, between covering for summer vacations and adding new functions to already busy employees. The accounting office is also overwhelmed with balancing out Visa/MasterCard machines daily. Thus, adding cash counting, verification and batching is time consuming. Hopefully, as we continue to work through the process, adjust staff roles and provide ongoing training we will see consistently improving results.

Section III: Trickles

Stray Pearls and Helpful Tactics

"Good entrepreneurs will generally make enough money to live comfortably. But outstanding entrepreneurs are those who desire to live extravagantly."

Peter Drucker

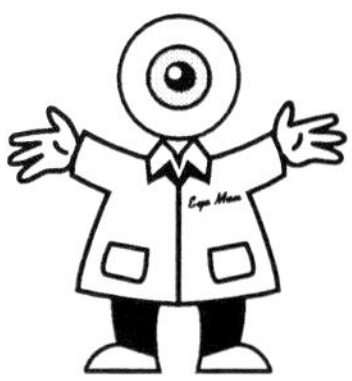

We've provided in this last, short section a miscellaneous selection of some of those tricks and trade secrets that ophthalmic practice management veterans have developed through the years to stay ahead of the pack. Some of these tactics didn't fit conveniently in the main body of the text. Some of these tactics are discussed in one way or another in other parts of this book, but are so important that we wanted to make sure you read about them at least twice. These are not organized in any particular order, but are presented below for your random exploration and discovery. A much wider collection of practice pearls can be found in the expanded third edition of *John Pinto's Little Green Book of Ophthalmology*, available from ASOA.

Check Your Bank Statements For Daily Deposit Postings

Here's a simple cross-check to make sure that funds coming into the practice are being rapidly deposited. Pull out your most recent monthly bank account statement. Go to the deposits section. In a large clinic, you should see daily bank deposits. In smaller practices, you should have at least a deposit every other day. It's not unusual to examine the bank statements of otherwise well-run practices and see just one large deposit every week or two. This hold-up in cash flow is easy to overcome—simply establish rules for how often you run to the bank.

Put Your Money to Work

It's a small matter, especially with the current low interest rates, but make sure your practice checking account is interest bearing or is transferred daily to a separate money market account. For the typical mid-sized practice averaging $100,000 or more in their working account, this can amount to $2000 or more in added income each year.

Banks That Come to You

In a very few settings, where banks are highly competitive with each other, you may be able to find a financial institution that is willing to come to you to pick up your deposits, either for free or for a very nominal cost. This can save significant staff time (as a "quick run to the bank" stretches into two or three other personal errands). It can also improve security and safety in practices that operate in areas with higher crime rates.

What's an Appropriate Line of Credit?

A line of credit is a pre-negotiated credit facility signed with your bank to provide working and other capital for foreseen needs. Think of it as another kind of insurance policy, which should be "taken out" in the context of your practice's unique needs, and the other kind of conventional insurance you already have. You obviously don't need a line of credit if you are independently wealthy and don't mind putting your own capital into the business. You may also not need a line of credit if you have a small practice and lots of business continuation insurance (in the event of your temporary disability) or have an extremely large practice, with many hands covering the monthly bills in case your personal production is knocked out for a time. But for the average practice, to get through times of normal stress (payer hiccups, unexpected absences from the practice, expected bubbles of expenditure on new projects), it's appropriate to negotiate one or more lines of credit equaling not less than three-month's expenses. For a practice with $1 million in annual collections and a 60 percent cost margin—or $50,000 a month in expenses—this would be a line of credit of at least $150,000. Obviously, like a home equity loan on your house, this should be negotiated well before you need it, tapped sparingly, and used only when other resources are unavailable.

Aging Report Accuracy

Aging, or "aged trial balance" (ATB) reports should be run based on the date of service, not the date of charge posting. A billing department that generates the latter kind of ATB report unwittingly makes it appear that cash flow is better than it actually is. Also, in many systems, refiling a claim will set the aging clock back. We've been to offices where the billing managers (with some guile) have rigged the reports so that the office appears to be very current in its accounts receivable management. You'll never know how polished your billing department is until you ask the right question: "Do you age by date of service or charge posting?"

An Annual Amnesty Program

When a patient owes the doctor a small amount of money, the patient is in trouble—when the patient owes a great amount of money, it's the doctor who's in trouble. The pearl that follows may not sit right with every practice, but it may be helpful in your setting. Some clinics have a soft heart, and as a result, every year they gather patients who still haven't paid their bills despite multiple demand letters, and they have not yet sent these patients to collections (which they probably should have much earlier.) Before sending these patients to collections (or in lieu of that if you're really a softie) you can send out a last letter that states that if patients in arrears pay just X percent of their bills by December 31st, the balance of their bills will be waived in the spirit of the holiday season.

Should We Add Cosmetic Surgery?

On the face of it, intuitively, providing cosmetic surgery should be a great way to augment cash flow for a practice. But experience shows it's very difficult for the typical ophthalmologist to add elective plastic surgery to his practice, for a variety of reasons. First and foremost, most surgeons are uncomfortable being as pushy as it takes to help a patient who has come in to see better understand that there are other services available. Vision care deals largely with *objective*, measurable improvements. Both the doctor and the patient are convinced that there's been a great operative outcome. Cosmetic surgery depends on the patient's *subjective* impression that the operation has been a success. If you do not currently provide cosmetic surgery and think you might be good at the promotional aspects, start first with botox injections. The barrier to entry is low, and you'll learn quickly if you can deal with three patients a morning who say, "I think we're a-l-m-o-s-t there…could we try some more?"

Examine Your Cataract Operative Criteria

Pull up charts of the last 50 cataract surgeries you've performed. Write down the best-corrected pre-operative visual acuity for each eye. Now average the resulting 50 numbers. If you're an aggressive surgeon, your average figure may come out somewhere in the 20/40-20/50 range. If you're much more conservative, your average figure may fall well over 20/80. Obviously, the cash flow and profits of cataract surgeons with the lower average number is going to be more favorable—to a point. Get too aggressive, and you may one day find yourself working backward in the cash flow department, refunding fees to payers for unnecessary surgery. If you're too conservative, due to age or personal skills deficits, it may be time to link up with a more accomplished surgeon for the benefit of both your patients and your pocketbook.

What Problem Do We Have Today?

Think about it. There are fundamentally only two kinds of business problems:

- Capacity Problems: The practice has more patients than capacity to see them. More doctors, staff or facilities are needed—or the resources you have must be better used.

- Volume Problems: The practice doesn't have enough business. So we need more marketing, diversification into new niche markets, or, as a last resort, we need to shed excess capacity.

Most growing practices move sequentially through cycles. They have excess capacity so they market or rekindle recall efforts. Then they have excess volume, so they add a doctor, and the cycle starts over again.

Prepare For the Cash Flow Consequences of Any Proposed Action Before You Act

If such analysis indicates you may be treading financial water for awhile, you must assure in advance your access to any needed capital. Here's a common example: A two-surgeon practice hires a new subspecialist. There are immediate costs for marketing, equipment, and generally setting up a new nest for the doctor. Then problems hit. There's a clerical snafu or a holdup in securing a Medicare provider number. Or credentialing for managed care contracts is slow in coming. In situations like this, especially in a low profit margin practice, carrying a new associate can make it hard to make payroll for the existing doctors. The time to go to your banker to negotiate a bridge loan or line of credit is before you need the money.

Are You Ready for Complexity?

If you aim to make your business larger or more diverse, you must be prepared to manage the resulting complexities. Even small, simple, solo practices have lots of moving parts and squeaking wheels. This enterprise complexity grows logarithmically with scale. You and your management team should master your current practice first. In the case of a merger or acquisition, you hardly have any right to run another doctor's practice if you have not yet mastered your own company.

What's an Accretive Decision?

Every practice initiative should, within an acceptable timeframe, be accretive to the net earnings of every owner. That's just a fancy way of saying that your business decisions should be made with the aim of eventually resulting in more profit per hour per owner doctor. Let's take an example: In a five-surgeon practice, Dr. Smith's pod is going to be built out with two more exam rooms at a cost of $75,000, charged evenly to the partnership. On the surface, it seems like Smith is getting a great deal and his partners are hosed, right? Wrong. If in the next year Dr. Smith uses these rooms to produce another $300,000 in collections, both Smith and his partners will get a pay raise; Smith gets the money directly as a producer, of course, but he and his partners also get an indirect benefit by having more of their fixed overhead covered. Following this rule doesn't promise that every doctor will get an *equal* benefit from every development decision, but that every doctor will be better off at the end of the day.

What's in it For....E-V-E-R-Y-B-O-D-Y?

When developing, you must align the incentives for all of the stakeholders in your practice. Fair enough: As a surgeon-owner, it's reasonable for you to ask first, "What's in it for me?" But immediately after this you should also ask, "What do my partners get? What do staff members get? What does the doctor whose practice I merge with get?" If the incentives are markedly unbalanced, your plan may be destined to failure.

Remember: Healthcare is a Local Business.

Don't over-extend your supply lines to distant operations unless you have abundant capital and proven operational competence. For most surgeons, staking out satellite operations more than 25 miles away without planting a homeroom doctor in the subject market is becoming a very dis-economic business model as fees continue to erode and practice costs continue to rise. Try to have the discipline to remember that success should be measured in profit per surgeon-hour (including travel time), not cases per month.

It's Not Case Volumes But Profits That Count

Many surgeons with the highest case volumes don't take home the largest paychecks. And while they may be among the most driven doctors, they certainly aren't always the happiest. By the time you back out optometric co-management fees and the marketing costs needed to drive a top-tier practice, the annual income hero in your town may be someone you least suspect, especially when calculated on a profit-per-hour basis.

Icing on the Patient Encounter Cake

A very few, select practices send follow up letters to their patients after the first visit (or even after every visit) thanking them for coming in and dropping in a customized or canned paragraph abstracting how the visit went. The paragraph reads something like this: "As you know you have the early signs of cataract formation in your eye. I don't believe that this appreciably impacts your vision yet. But together, in the months and years ahead, let's monitor these cataract changes. I can assure you that when the time comes, we will be able to treat your cataracts effectively and comfortably using the latest methods."

Filling the Seats

Here's a great pearl for doctors who still can't quite seem to get their staff to fully book out the appointment template—they have patients booked out a month, but tomorrow's calendar has 48 slots and only 43 are filled. It's deceptively simple. For every day that the template is filled 100 percent with appointments (before no-shows peel this back) every staff member (in a small office) or selected staff (in a larger practice) get a $5-10 bonus. That may seem excessive. But do the math. Let's say it's a small 12-staff office. Five patients are gained in this case. The average ticket might be $150. That's $750. And almost all of it is profit, because it's incremental revenue and generates no additional fixed overhead. The cost? Twelve staff times let's say $8 would total just $96. And the resulting morale boost also is worth the cost alone. Doing this is probably the only way in the world you'll ever get techs going to the front desk and pestering your clerks in the afternoon, saying, "Are you sure we can't fit a few more patients on the schedule for the morning?"

Be Sure to Take Your Charm Pills Every Morning

We've seen more great practices with technically great surgeons bite the dust because the surgeons just were not very charming to patients (or staff.) We've seen a number of technically lackluster surgeons and practices, offering so-so care to the public, but doing so at high volumes because the doctors were charming. There are obvious cash flow advantages to acting "nice," even if you have to fake it. If you can't turn it around, or be completely nice, then at least work on not making everyone mad at you at the same time.

Choices Enhance Profits

Mediocre administrators will give their managers or their boards ultimatums: "We must do this!" Exceptional managers give the people they supervise, and those to whom they are subordinate, two or more equally acceptable alternatives: "I've brought three alternate plans for us to consider today. I believe that any one of these that you choose can solve the problem we've been wrestling. If, as a manager, you force yourself to come up with at least two or three viable solutions to problems that land on your desk, chances are you'll at least double the odds of finding the best and most profitable solution.

Back Up Your Manager

Remember back to grammar school or perhaps high school. Can you recall all those deliciously cruel days when you had a substitute teacher? And almost without active coordination the entire class worked as a team to undercut the sub's authority? It can be the same way in your practice if you have one or more doctors who undercut the authority of your administrator. The manager of your practice needs to be the "real teacher" not the "substitute."

Optical Profits Increasingly Vital to Practice Survival

The relationship between a general ophthalmology practice and its optical is a little like the relationship between a fine restaurant and its bar. A significant percentage of the profits come from the optical. Those profits are passive, requiring little additional work from the "chef" who's back in the "kitchen." When the clinic ("restaurant") is overflowing, the optical ("bar") is a nice place for patrons to hang out. Optical goods complement what's on the clinic's main menu. In optometry, optical provides virtually all of the practice's profits. Although never to the same extent, we think this will be increasingly the case in ophthalmology.

Beware Optical Discount Plans

The typical ophthalmic optical dispensary generates a 20-25 percent profit margin. Typical optical discount plans reduce your top line 10-20 percent. Therefore, it can be dangerous—even if you're trying to drive incremental revenue or cross-sell managed care patients to elective surgical care—to sign up with discount optical plans.

Medicaid Optical and Medical Payment Trends

In an apparently increasing number of states, Medicaid patients and their providers are forced to outsource optical goods from their care provider to central vendors. In such states, the doctor gets a token service fee to dispense glasses. This is unfortunate, since optical profits have often been one of the last remaining incentives for accepting Medicaid patients, along with a spike in the recent past—in selected states—in fee payments secondary to the tobacco settlements. Now that a large number of states are running budget deficits with a downturn in the economy, Medicaid money is on the chopping block. In California, as this book goes to press, a 15 percent reduction in MediCal (California's version of Medicaid) is proposed, along with a massive disenrollment of fringe beneficiaries. It seems clear that all health reimbursement signs, public sector and private, point to sharp curtailments unless an unexpected and robust turnaround in the general economy surfaces. Strong provider efficiency and work ethic, increased patient volumes, and cost containment will have to harmonize to allow personal income stasis, much less growth, for the average ophthalmologist.

Graphing Your Performance For Better Practice Analysis

Tracking monthly surgical cases, clinic visits, charges, receivables, and a host of other volume performance data is a critical part of the regular business analysis you should be performing in today's rapidly changing environment. Some surgeons and managers can glance down columns of figures and immediately spot what's going on. But most of us mortals do a better job spotting trends when we can see the data graphically.

A Quick Visual Audit of Technician Productivity

It's sometimes hard to know if all of the practice's technicians are working at the same pace. The surgeon-employer is dashing from room to room. The tech supervisor is as likely to be working up patients as watching traffic on the floor. And office managers who come from a business background can be shy about critiquing tech productivity. Simply hand each tech a different colored highlighter pen. And keep a separate printout of the day's patients back at the nurses' station. As each tech starts a patient, they mark that patient in their personalized color. The doctor and senior tech can look at the printed schedule at the end of each day and rapidly see who's doing what. Over several days , it's easy to see who is cherry-picking the quick checks and who is working double-time.

Health Insurance Fact Sheets

Patients show up at the front desk daily with questions about their insurance. They're often confused about what benefits they enjoy and the process they must undergo to take full advantage of these benefits. Like as not, they blame you and your practice for oversights or coverage gaps, instead of their carriers. It all takes a toll on staff time, efficiency, and morale. Here's a partial solution: Make up simple fact sheets on the most common payers in your service area, and perhaps one generic sheet to cover all the rest. Taking pains in writing to explain what co-pays and deductibles and refraction fees are all about will have several positive benefits. It will educate patients and hopefully make them a little more understanding of your role. It increases consistency and reduces the chance that an uninformed staffer will misguide a patient. It will save staff time and hassle factor—they can handle the more elaborate or customized questions. And it will likely lead to less resistance to cover their patient-responsible amounts at checkout.

Great Billing Advice May Be Just Down the Street

One of the least expensive and most effective sources for help with billing problems are staff in regional eye care practices just like yours. You and Dr. Jones may compete vigorously, and it would not be likely to find your marketing departments collaborating—but it's very useful to develop relationships between patient accounts departments. It may even be helpful to formalize this with periodic group meetings to share pearls related to local carrier challenges. What's especially useful, is if you can network with practices that have your same computer system. One caveat, however. Just because Mary Jane from the neighboring practice says that something is correct, does not necessarily make it so. The higher the stakes, the more you should cross-check multiple sources.

Physician and Staff Computer Literacy

Every practice, irrespective of size, should have at least two key operators for their computer system capable of handling all routine operations and report writing, and moderate levels of troubleshooting. Without this precaution, your cash flow could come to an abrupt halt if you lost just one key worker. The more geographically remote the practice, the more important these skills become. In addition, the managing physician partner of a practice (at the very least) should have the ability to use the system. The administrator (at least) should have access to an on-line service and be comfortable performing research work on the internet.

Computer Conversion Tip

When making a conversion to a new computer system, it's intelligent to keep the old system up and running...and not just to collect old accounts. Run a few trial electronic claims on the new system first. Work out the bugs. Depending on your vendor selection, these may be minimal, and you can immediately plow ahead after the test runs and leave the old system far behind. But on the off chance that you have major conversion difficulties, this backup could save a lot of headaches. This may seem like common sense advice, but many practices have ditched their old systems before their new system was properly tested and had to scramble instead of solving their conversion problems in leisure. Remember, it's not your computer and it's your cash flow.

A Checklist for Selecting a New Practice Computer System

- Do you even need an entirely new system, or an upgrade of your present system? Make sure that the requirement for a new system is driven by real needs (the core of which are to preserve and improve patient accounts management) and not a doctor's passing fancy.
- Do you have sufficient expertise resident within the practice to interview vendors and make a purchase decision?
- Do you have an in-house key operator? If you are upgrading to a more robust system with paperless charting, inventory and other chores beyond A/R management and scheduling, you may need a dedicated information system director.
- Have you factored into your transition costs the staff frustrations, staff overtime and likely cash-flow interruption? Do you have capital reserves set aside to cover worst-case transition scenarios?
- Are you allowing enough time to make a wise decision?
- Are you budgeting enough? A typical, basic small office system from a major vendor now runs $50,000 or more.
- Are you budgeting too much? An overly sophisticated system will only add friction to your practice's training program and ultimately impede cash flow.
- Have you seen the contemplated system successfully installed and hard at work in at least three practices comparable to yours? Have you talked first-hand with staff in these practices?
- Does your contemplated system have a large enough user base? Newer or localized systems may have just a few users, and be dependent on a single key guru at the home office. Lose the guru, and you start over again.
- Is there sufficient customer support in the home office? Ask a minimum of five ophthalmic users who have been using your contemplated system for more than a year for their assessment of response time, effectiveness and patience levels.
- Have I had a side-by-side live demonstration of all finalist systems we're contemplating? Nothing will make a salesperson more honest and more price-competitive than having their peers in the same room.

- Is there a satisfaction guarantee? Will your vendor take back the system within 6 months, no questions asked, if you don't like it?

It's Not "Worth" if It's Not Put to "Work"

Billing and coding consulting firms take pains to research your practice's patterns, and write up their findings. But as the Chinese proverb says, "To know, and not to do, is not to know." Make sure that such reports don't just sit on the administrator's desk, but that the principle findings get shared with all relevant parties on a need-to-know basis. Note that sometimes the contents of these reports is highly sensitive, so the entire report should not simply be passed around to all hands. However, make sure that any reasonable suggestions for policy changes are the basis for re-writing your protocols, and scheduling appropriate auditing and training sessions.

"Do We Have ALL of Your Insurance Information?"

A significant amount of re-work is done in every insurance department, chasing down blind alleys for payment. You can eliminate some of this by making sure that the front desk always inquires of patients about their co-payer status, makes copies of all insurance card changes. It's frustrating to bill the incorrect secondary payer, and then have to start all over again with a new payer. This points out, once again, the value of having the patient accounts and front desk staff under a single department head, so that problems in one area can be smoothly resolved in a contributing area.

Inspect What You Expect

It makes anyone nervous to have a supervisor hovering around ready to pounce on errors. That's why it's not only more effective, but more humane, to let your staff know—in writing—what performance you expect. Make it clear that charges for the day's services should be posted by the end of the same service day, or by noon the following day, or whatever your policy calls out. It's not fair to hold people accountable for occult policies and procedures. Write it down…train to what's written…then inspect at will.

Are You a Fast or Slow Technology Adopter?

Every practice likes to think of itself as leading edge, up on the latest knowledge and at the ready to provide the latest services to patients, right? Well, like every other part of your practice, it's a question of balance. Unless you work in a setting supported by unlimited grant monies, you have to pick and choose as new technologies and techniques arrive. Too liberal a policy, and you could spend hundreds of thousands of dollars a year on gadgets, many with doubtful clinical application or financial rationale in your setting. We've seen practices (an increasing number, unfortunately) sink under the weight of too rapid an adoption curve. But the opposite, using the same old rattle-trap equipment year after year, is just as damaging to a practice, and to the quality of patient care. Ask yourself and trusted colleagues, "Are we too fast, too slow, or just right in our technology adoption pace?" In general, most ophthalmologists are weighted toward the former, and their administrators have to put their foot down around the time of the national meetings.

It's Not Your Phone, It's Your Business

In the voicemail world we've all gritted our teeth and become accustomed to, and with rising staff costs, it's not unusual for practices to succumb to the trap of having a skeleton phone staff and resorting to messages on hold for callers. Don't do it. Ophthalmology is best and most profitably performed with as much of the human touch as possible. Resorting to the false economy of automated appointment reminder calls is similarly ineffective. Our experience in the field is that practices using automated calling for appointment reminders have their no-show rates increase 50 percent to 100 percent. Norms are a 5 percent no-show rate in most general/suburban practices. In a practice where staff and doctors see 50 patients a day, that's two or three patients a day. The loss of an extra two or three patients, by using a computer rather than even a very junior clerk to call, results in a +/- $350 in lost revenue for the day. A clerk can rescue this by getting the calling job done in 60-80 minutes at a cost of about $20, including phone charges and floor space. Not a bad return on investment.

Read Provider Contracts Before Signing... Then Keep Checking

Don't assume you have to accept every contract that comes across your desk just as it's written. If you have any kind of negotiating position (you don't really need the patients, the payment level is borderline, or the payer is notoriously late in paying) consider coming back with suggested changes to speed or increase payments, or reduce paperwork. And do make sure, to the extent possible, that every contract has a fee schedule attached, even if this can be changed at a whim by most payers. Periodically, ask for updated fee schedules and compare your actual payments per the EOB with this fee schedule to assure that you are still being paid per the contracted allowable.

Spread Payables Duties Around to Ward Off Diversion

It's not unusual, especially in smaller practices, to have one office manager or bookkeeper review vendor invoices, write the checks (even sign or stamp them!), prepare the general ledger and profit and loss statements, and *also* reconcile the bank statements each month. This clearly leaves open many opportunities for embezzlement. A doctor (the same one each month for consistency) should sign all checks above trivial amounts (let's say $250-500) which can be signed by the office manager. Checks ready for signature should be attached to the relevant invoice, and the purchase agent or other person who can verify the bill should have signed off the invoice. The monthly general ledger (showing all checks as a separate line item, arranged according to your chart of account e.g. "utilities") should be reviewed by the doctor. Any unusual-sounding vendors should be asked about. Reconciliation of the bank statement to the general ledger should typically be performed by the practice's outside accountant, as another safeguard against diversion.

Monthly Financial Statements

In the bygone era of small, simple practices with 60 percent profit margins, "checkbook accounting" was sufficient—just by keeping track of the balance in your operating account, you knew enough to make most management decisions. Anyway, a 5 percent or 10 percent management mistake wasn't so critical. That era is no more. Profit margins of 40 percent and lower are quite normal today, and 15 percent-25 percent urban practice profits may not be out of the ordinary in just a few years. For doctor-owners, especially, it's time to get intimate with the month-by-month details of your practice. Some pointers:

- You should receive a cash basis income statement at least by the 20th of every month. An increasing number of practices generate their own statements in-house using QuickBooks, or any of the other numerous user-friendly computer programs now available (most smaller practices should avoid more powerful accounting programs which are designed for more complex enterprises).
- Your monthly statement should have columns showing (a) the current month's performance, (b) year-to-date figures (with each chart-of-account line item of expense broken out as a percentage of collections), and at least last year's year-to-date comparison.
- Better organized and larger practices will typically develop a department-by-department or overall practice budget forecast and then compare this budget to actual performance.

- Physician owners too often skip over the financial statements and go straight to the monthly compensation worksheet. The practice's administrator or accountant should act as a tutor and provide their doctors with an external source of discipline to study the numbers every month. Some spoon-feeding can help. Consider adding a brief narrative to every monthly statement:

  > "For the ten-month period ending October 31 compared to last year, charges were up 10 percent, but collections were down 4 percent due in equal parts to larger contractual allowances and our staff still adjusting to the computer upgrade. Expenses were up 15 percent, largely due to Dr. Smith's self-insured malpractice settlement and a continued ramp up of marketing. Payroll costs have fallen somewhat as we have done a better job controlling overtime. Dr. Jones's growing plastic surgery practice is keeping ahead of our loss of senior patients to capitated plans."

- If you generate income statements in-house, they should be reviewed at least quarterly or semiannually by your accountant to facilitate tax planning. Many practices generate a trial statement, and hand this preliminary document to their accountant for refinement (along with routine chores like bank statement reconciliation.)

Cash Basis Accounting

Generally speaking, there are two ways to prepare profit and loss statements for your practice. Accrual basis accounting counts revenue when you charge for your services and counts expenses when you receive an invoice. It's a terrific system for manufacturing and retail environments, where the time cycle between taking delivery on raw or wholesale goods and their eventual sale as finished goods or retail products can be stretched out for months or quarters. But accrual accounting is ill-suited to ambulatory health care, including eye care services. Cash basis accounting provides the most meaningful snapshot of practice health: Revenue is counted when collected and expenses are counted when paid.

When Should I Pay This Bill?

The answer is, "It depends." You should certainly pay it no earlier than it is due. And you may want to stretch out payment as long as possible if your practice is in a cash flow bind (as increasingly happens in the first quarter of the year, even in well-run practices.) On the other hand, you want to secure every possible discount by paying early. Any "2 percent net 10 day" accounts (where you subtract 2 percent from the bill for paying early) should obviously be paid within the 10-day window.

We're all familiar with the concept of aging your receivables to have some sense of where the practice stands on collecting outstanding accounts. It's much less common in a service sector business like ophthalmology, where most trade payables are paid within 10-45 days, to age your payables. But this is exactly what you should start doing if and when you find yourself in any financial tight spot, to the point of having to start stretching out vendor payments. Don't be like the administrator who hid a sheaf of invoices from the doctor just to make the books look good and achieve the number that equated a bonus.

Understand Your Ability to Say, "No Thanks"

"Walk-away power," as in having the power to walk away from a bad deal, is an old term for a common sense concept. If, as a customer, you have one or more alternative vendors, the advantage is in your court. If you can buy elsewhere you have the advantage. If you don't have to buy right away, you have the advantage. Always think in terms of what your alternatives are if the negotiations fail. Can you wait a few months and try again? At the very least, even if you only have one choice in vendors and you need delivery NOW, conduct negotiations as if you have a viable fallback position.

What's the Real Price?

Don't ever be too embarrassed to ask for a discount. The worst that can happen is that the vendor will decline—but may then unconsciously make efforts to shave charges the next time a bid is delivered, knowing you're cost-sensitive. Here's a simple new habit you can start tomorrow—a core secret of the very rich that will save you bundles both professionally and personally:

Always ask for a better price, even in unexpected places, like retail stores, where all the prices are marked. This is difficult, even embarrassing, for many people (including your spouse, if you really get into this). So here is some scripting to get you started:

- "I'd like to buy this, but the price is more than I'm willing to pay. Is there anything you can do to adjust the price?";
- "I have a friend who might also want to order one of these—what discount could we get buying two?";
- "If you can't lower the price any further, are there any accessories you can throw in?";
- "What's the lowest price at which you sell these?";

- "Is there a discount available for paying with cash?";
- "I'm sure I've seen these for a lot less—is there anything you can do on the price for me today?";
- "I can't tell you who for obvious reasons, but I know that a colleague of mine buys these from your company for a lot lower price than what you're offering me.";
- "I'm torn between your product and your competitor's, so now we're just down to price. What's the lowest you can sell this for and still make a fair profit?"; and
- "Is the price for this going to come down?"

Cutting Utility Costs

Here are tips to reduce lighting and power costs:

- Update your thermostat for a timed unit rather than keeping the temperature stable at all hours;
- Relocate work stations that need more light. Group them in areas with more natural illumination, if available;
- Campaign to turn off the lights when they're not needed;
- Install high-efficiency fluorescent lights;
- If you design a new building or an addition or consider taking on a larger lease, reduce space needs to the greatest possible extent; and
- Color-code light switches, showing which should be on at all times, which should be on during working hours, which should only be on for after-hours maintenance workers.

Should My Practice Be Audited By Our Accountant?

Periodic deep or even shallow auditing of the practice's books by an outside accountant is an often-overlooked area of good practice management hygiene. This need not include the full green eye shades treatment but just a half day snooping around once or twice a year. The key value that emerges from this review is physician peace of mind. The secondary gains include a) staff know that someone will look over their shoulders periodically, so their work tends to be a bit neater and any thoughts of larceny are dampened, and b) as you grow, your accountant—by orbiting more closely—will be in a position to suggest improvements in funds flow through the organization.

Trust But Check

Daily, or at least on a frequent spot audit basis, someone in the practice should audit the appointment schedule, patient sign-in sheet, charts, super bills and laser log and comparing these to the charge ledgers. Missed charges for services provided are common and amount to tens of thousands or more in lost revenues per year in the typical practice—lost profits and ruined cash flow.

Doctors: Ask For Feedback

Most staff, even the sassiest, are shy about going to their doctors and pointing out their faults. This can lead to serious cash flow hiccups. Taking their advice with an open mind could markedly improve practice profits. You should publicly and frequently ask your staff to give you feedback. This can either be direct and face-to-face or can be anonymous. The most common suggestions they'll make will most likely include:

- Come to the office on time and get right to work instead of dawdling;
- Fill out the superbill correctly every time;
- Act cheerful and not as if we've interrupted you when we need a signature or clarification;
- Don't take personal calls when we're behind;
- Stop giving out excess courtesy discounts or free care to people you barely know;
- Don't pick out staff favorites and give them special treatment;
- Don't pick on the people over and over, and don't do so publicly or out of all proportion to the offense;
- Don't roll your eyes, pout, or tell us, "It must be kill the doctor day." Your staff really are trying their level best to make it a great practice;
- In most cases, don't have your spouse work in the practice, unless she/he is so competent they could hold the same job in another practice; and
- Act positive, and especially provide positive reinforcement to areas of the practice you don't work in, such as insurance.

Every Financial Tool Should Agree

Your practice has a number of financial tools to measure volume performance, collections and cash flow. You likely have an appointment module and can cross-correlate this to any missing fee slips/superbills for the day, which should in turn tie to posted charges and patient-responsible amounts received on that day, charges, collections, bank statements (and their reconciliation) all of which should eventually tie with the profit and loss statement for the practice and it's various operating segments. These various tools should be closed out at the same time, to the extent possible, and in agreement. Only a minority of practices actually tie their disparate financial reports together in this fashion. Those that do can immediately spot sloppy entries and inappropriate write-offs.

Track the Volatility of Your Average Collections, Average Charges and Other Graphs

You may not pay particular attention to the financial details, but you can at least grossly monitor the stability of your practice's financial pulse by graphing each month, or 24 months or more, the monthly collections and charges divided by the number of patient visits. Obviously, the average charge per patient will be more stable than the average collections per patient visit because in the latter case, you are collecting for services rendered 30 to 60 days or longer ago. However, any excess swings and volatility in these graphs that are not explained by similar wide swings in vacation time are warning signs that should be tracked down to their source.

"Payer, May I?"

It's a very complex variation on the children's game, "Mother may I," that managed care payers play with doctors and their staff. Lack of referral and treatment authorization leads to untracked millions of dollars in lost fees to ophthalmologists annually. In the hum and flow of the typical urban practice, it's not practical, nor expected that you will win the game 100 percent of the time. Just like back in kindergarten, you are going to lose concentration and slip up on occasion. The best remedy is to have sufficient staff and sufficient training to be able to cover the best efforts of payers to not pay (which is of course the way that *they* win the game.) Like any game, you need to have and study a copy of the rules. You need to make sure that all the players know the rules. And every time you lose the game by slipping up, you need to huddle with the rest of the players on your team, know how many points you've just lost, and run through the ways this can be prevented in the future. That's the generic advice, at least. Obviously, the regional variations on this frustrating game is something you simply have to learn by experience in your own setting. When in doubt, always check. Create a grid by payer, memorized by all staff and doctors, showing what services are allowed by what providers in your practice, after what pre-authorization steps are taken. Always be suspicious of payers you don't serve often. And along the way, be sure to keep the patient (the unfortunate pawn in this game) as educated as possible. Unfortunately, unless otherwise informed, they are going to blame you, not their carrier, for any limitations on their access to your services.

Did This Test Really Happen?

Biometry, visual field and similar testing equipment that print out results should be checked periodically to make sure that the printed reports reflect the correct date. Failure to show the correct date, in the event of an audit, could lead to some embarrassing explanations as to why the chart date conflicts with the print-out date. Add this to your monthly or weekly checklist in the office.

Are you Sure?

A similar "picky, picky detail" problem can occur with special tests that require follow up reporting or interpretation by the ordering doctor. If this reporting is absent from the chart, then the relevant service cannot be billed. Develop a protocol in your office to make sure that all special testing has been subsequently interpreted. This can be done by comparing the written log for the special testing equipment (or the patient accounts print-out) with the contents of each subject chart. If periodic audits show you follow up 100 percent of the time, you can reduce the audit frequency. If your practice has an intractable problem with this, it may help to establish a routine where all special testing printouts destined for interpretation are clipped or stapled to the front of the chart, and not filed away until the interpretation is completed.

More Detail Work to Catch Billing Gaps

It's quite easy, in the heat of battle, to forget to document special testing or treatment on the superbill. Here are a couple of quick cross-audits. First, the number of ultrasounds should be roughly the same as the number of cataract surgeries in any one month. Second, every unit of testing and treatment equipment should have a use log showing date, patient name and appropriate utilization records. If you compare the gross number of YAG lasers on the log for last month, with the number of YAGs charged out in the same timeframe, the numbers should match exactly.

Getting Paid For a Needed Patient Service

On what portion of your cataract surgical patients do you perform intraoperative or postoperative relaxing incisions? Although new lens materials and smaller incisions have markedly reduced induced astigmatism, a small percent of patients go to cataract surgery with innate astigmatism, the correction of which will not be reimbursed by Medicare. You can approach such patients with the option of performing limbal relaxing incisions at a typical cost of as much as $300 per eye.

Differential Collection Ratios as a Marker for Billing Snafus

In a multi-physician practice, it may be very revealing to look at the collection ratio by doctor. Of course, there will be an expected variance based on practice patterns and patient mix. Pediatric ophthalmologists and LASIK surgeons in the same practice will have markedly different ratios for obvious reasons. But for two general ophthalmologists/cataract surgeons in the same practice, the collection ratio should be essentially the same. When it's not, look for both the obvious and the subtle disparities. Is one doctor the sole contractor for a low-paying contract? Or does one doctor's behaviors (like hoarding charts after surgery and not dictating or coding the case for several weeks) explain the difference. One source of this kind of problem that we've seen is when the patient accounts team gives the senior doctor's accounts the VIP treatment because he signs their checks. In turn, they pay less attention to the open accounts of junior doctors. Harness the natural competitive feelings within a practice to optimize everyone's revenue yield.

Options to 100 percent ASC Development and Ownership

What should you do if you don't have the necessary cataract case volumes or risk tolerance or management coverage to develop your own surgery center? There are basically three options:

1. You can join in the syndication of a group ASC. This may be an ophthalmic-only center or a multi-specialty center. Your costs and risks will be much lower, but keep in mind that your returns are likely to be lower, too, in percentile terms especially with a multi-specialty center. Such facilities typically have only a 15-25 percent profit margin compared with dedicated eye ASCs at 35+ percent.

2. You can turn to a development/management company such as NovaMed or AmSurg to carry the ball. This allows you to own (and be responsible for) half or less of a facility and may help to diffuse difficult local politics of bringing other partners into the deal.

3. You can rent facilities and staff by the day from an appropriate local facility and have the benefits of your own private space, but with no investment outlays or capital at risk. This approach can be a potential bridge to developing your own dedicated facility (when your numbers slowly rise). In this instance, there is no non-compete agreement in place, as there would be with options 1 and 2.

HMO v. Indemnity Economics

In fee-for-service medicine, we need to concentrate on revenue enhancement (marketing, building surgical density) because most costs are fixed and profits soar rapidly after a minimal volume threshold is reached. In pre-paid medicine, our management emphasis turns to cost containment because our revenue for a given block of lives under contract is fixed. A significant squeeze is experienced by most HMO-heavy practices when patients demand more services, payers demand per-member-per-month fee concessions and inflation inexorably raises expenses.

Basic Capitation Contract Caveats

As this book goes to press, capitation contracting continues to wane for ophthalmology and for Medicare beneficiaries. Strong pockets of pre-paid care continue to hold on in selected markets, and one can forecast that with health costs continuing to escalate at a double-digit pace, some HMO-like products will find their way back onto the market and into your billing office. Here are some very basic issues and warnings related to such contracts:

- Look carefully before leaping. What may seem like a great way to trump the competition may end up leaving them time and the inclination to redouble efforts to get higher-paying patients;

- Review the covered services in the contract. Especially check to see if you will be responsible for subspecialty care. If so, and you don't have in-house subspecialists, the cost of such care with outside providers will be subtracted from your payments. This is an easy way to "blow your cap." Try, in most cases, to have outside subspecialty care paid for by the HMO directly;

- What starts as incremental income for your practice, for selling unused incremental time, can turn into major time commitments that edge out better-paying patients. Make sure that any one contract (except Medicare) never exceeds 15-25 percent of your total collections;

- It is typical for HMOs to withhold 10-20 percent of the capitation fee to cover any losses due to over-utilization. In evaluating your go/no-go with a potential contract, base your decision on the least amount that you are assured of receiving, not the most. You must also review the contract closely to assure that you will not be obliged to cover any over-utilization losses that exceed the withheld amounts;

- Beware of accepting pre-paid contracts for small beneficiary pools. The actuarial statistics work for large pools but break down with smaller groups of patients;

- Negotiate, if you can, capitation payment increases indexed to any increases in premiums charged by the HMO to employers;
- Capitation payments are made monthly, accompanied by a statement showing the number of beneficiaries. Watch this statement for adverse trends, especially any trends that reduce the beneficiary pool down to a size that invades the actuarial soundness of your capitation payment. Negotiate in advance if possible to be guaranteed a minimum number of assigned patients;
- Medicare cap rates are obviously higher—often 4-6+ times higher—than cap rates for commercial-aged patients due to the much higher utilization rates of older patients; and
- Remember that accepting your first capitation contract in a group practice obliges a close review of the compensation model. Compensation directly based on utilization (RVUs, visits, surgeries) will cause doctors to increase their utilization (in order to get a larger share of the cap fee pie), which decreases the profit per unit of service rendered. It's more rational to divide capitation fees based on assigned patients, so that each doctor's incentives (to not over treat) are aligned with the HMOs payment methodology.

Dividing Up Billing Office Duties

Patient accounts departments commonly divide their work into payers, with "Martha" handling Blue Cross, "Sam" handling Medicare, and so forth. While this can foster individual expertise, it leaves the practice vulnerable to the departure of any single staff member in the billing office. Depending on the size of your practice, it may be better to divide patients along alphabetical lines. This will force cross training and build in staff redundancy. Although this approach makes things a little harder for the supervisor and the staff, it's ultimately somewhat more protective of the continuity of the practice's cash flow.

Are Multiple Fee Schedules Allowed?

If you are a typical ophthalmic practice, most of your revenue comes from Medicare. Maintaining just one fee schedule for all payers generally works well. Keep your total fees about 20 percent-30 percent above allowable Medicare rates, but be sure that you match or exceed the fees paid by any commercial payers. If you receive 100 percent of any of your charged fees from Medicare, it may mean that Medicare's allowable fee is higher than your charge. Fee reviews should be annual to make sure you keep up with changes. Keep in mind that patients see your fee on their explanation of benefits statement and may misperceive your high fee as an attempt to overcharge Medicare. To avoid this, and to avoid large write-offs and an inflated A/R, some practices will have two fee schedules: One for Medicare and one for all other carriers.

Documentation Basics

The following is a basic documentation checklist, abstracted from a Medicare carrier newsletter. Compare this list to documentation standards in your own practice:

- Medicare expects documentation to be generated at the time of service or shortly thereafter;
- Delayed entries (within 24-48 hours) are permitted for clarification, error correction, or the addition of data not initially available;
- The medical record cannot be altered. Corrections must be lined out legibly, dated and initialed;
- Delayed written explanations cannot be used to retrospectively support services billed or their medical necessity;
- All entries must be legible to another reader to a degree that a meaningful review can be conducted; and
- All notes should be dated, preferably timed, and signed by the author; initials are acceptable in an office setting where the author can be easily identified by initials. If the initials or signature are not legible, a printed version should also be recorded.

When Should You Collect Co-Pays and Deductibles?

Each office we visit has strong opinions about when co-payments, deductibles, refraction fees, and any other patient responsible amounts should be collected. Most of this conforms to local custom, the experience of each practice and the policy to which your patients have been habituated. The most aggressive practices, especially those in rural southeastern markets where "tricking the doctor" seems to be a community past time, office managers get the money up front as often as they can, before patient is allowed to see a doctor. Any past-due amounts from prior visits are also collected with a vengeance. This may seem mercenary, but really is indicated in some settings. At the other, 'Yankee' end of the spectrum, there are practices that collect nothing at the time of service. Zip. They end up chasing after patients with three letters and a phone call for a $10 co-pay. In the average setting, both of these extremes are skipped in favor of payment at the time of check-out.

Refraction Fee Trends

It wasn't that long ago that only a minority of practices charged a refraction fee, or what they charged was more of a nuisance fee than a reasonable exchange for the value conveyed to the patient. Recently, that has changed. The typical refraction fees we see now are in the $18-25 range, and a few bold practices are charging in excess of $30. The highest priced practices report, somewhat cynically perhaps, "Whoever is going to complain about a refraction fee is going to complain, no matter what we charge. So we decided to charge a premium, which offsets fee cuts a bit, pays us a fee that induces us to provide a superior level of care, compensates us for the tongue-lashing we get from a very small number of patients. No one else seems to mind."

Give Yourself As Many Second Chances As Possible

We'll say it here, with some affection: Most practices and most surgeons really don't try very hard to *make the sale*. We're not trying to be negative. Nor, do we think our advice verges on the unprofessional. It's just that the gentility of the average surgeon (and by abstraction, their management team) is not in synch with the increasingly difficult cash flow environment we're in today. Here are just some examples:

- Practices that let patients walk their glasses prescriptions out the door without making follow up calls to learn why the patient didn't buy glasses in their dispensary, and to offer them a 30-day coupon for $25 dollars off to prove that you do the best job in town;
- Practices that send out information to prospective LASIK patients without then making a series of follow up calls to ask patients to take the next steps and have consultations; and
- Surgeons who send patients home with a pat on the shoulder, saying, "Well Mrs. Arnold, you think about that cataract surgery and call me if you have any follow up questions" instead of saying, "Well Mrs. Arnold, you think about that cataract surgery and in about a week I'll have my chief medical assistant Mary give you a call to answer any follow-up questions. Meanwhile, here's a free videocassette on cataract surgery you can share with your husband and daughter."

Comanagement Guidelines

Some of the largest and most profitable practices in America are those that have developed a large network of relationships with optometrists in their region. In such practices, it is common to find that 50 percent or more of such patients are comanaged. And in most settings, these relationships are completely above board, appropriate and ethical and ultimately beneficial to patients. However, comanagement can be a slippery slope, with strong incentives to bend the guidelines. We hope for some clarifications in this murky area in the future, but for now, consider that the rules *may* potentially be broken when:

- Comanagement is used as an incentive for getting referrals;
- A referring doctor demands comanagement and threatens to withhold referrals to surgeons who will not comanage;
- The referring doctor's sole purpose for the referral is to get the comanagement fee;
- A surgeon opts for comanagement, and does divide the fee without delegating the care to the comanaging doctor;
- The surgeon returns the patient to the referring doctor on a pre-arranged date, rather than one indicated by the status of the patient;
- The surgeon is directly paying the referring doctor for referrals; and
- A surgeon comanages all of his patients with other providers as a matter of policy and not on a case-by-case basis.

Aging Report Pearls

The standard vanilla-flavored aging report lumps all payers together and only has aging buckets for current, 30, 60, 90, and 120+ day accounts. Consider generating your reports by carrier so you can spot adverse trends associated with slow payers. Also, if your computer allows, consider expanding the buckets to allow 121-160 day and 161 and over categories. As a doctor-owner, or administrator, you should meet with your patient accounts' staff monthly. Ask about the status of individual patient line items. If your staff can recite from rote (or at least from their notation fields) the status of high-balance/older open accounts, you can have some assurance they're on top of the details.

Helping Your Billing Department

Practice billing departments are always swamped with patient calls after every batch of statements is mailed. You can reduce this burden somewhat by adding a supplemental "Frequently Asked Questions" insert to your bill (or printing this on the statement if space permits.)

What is a "New" Patient?

It all depends on how you use the data. In the world of practice marketing, a new patient is just what you would expect—a patient who has never been a customer before. However, with respect to reimbursement, Medicare defines a new patient as one who has not received services from you or another doctor of the same specialty within the same group practice within the past three years, which means you can bill for a new patient visit.

Learn in a Flash

Let's face it: Most patient accounts work is mind-numbingly dull. If marketing is the sizzle of practice management, billing work is little more than scrubbing the frying pan. But it's obviously equally or more important than marketing. So how can we best teach doctors, techs, and others in the practice who need to know coding and reimbursement details cold? It may help to develop a set of flash cards. These can be specific to the needs of your individual practice, and prepared at a simple or more complex level depending on the skills of your people. You can prepare a basic set for all staff, and more advanced versions for staff who need a higher level of mastery.

Portable Brains

Of course, no matter how much you study coding and charting and reimbursement, there are going to be dark corners that you never commit to memory, especially if you don't work with billing daily. Consider laminating in plastic one or more cards with a "cheat sheet" of relevant details that can be kept handy in a lab coat pocket, and refreshed periodically.

Appendix One

Quick Checklist of Effective Office Tools

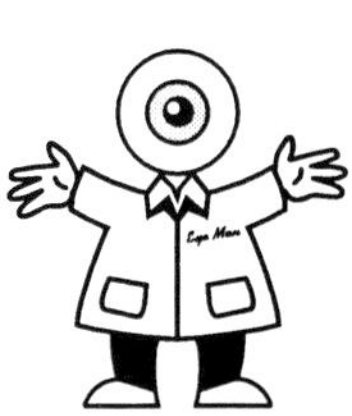

QUICK CHECKLIST OF EFFECTIVE OFFICE TOOLS

- Current CPT Coding Manual.
- Current ICD-9-CM Diagnosis Coding Manual.
- Medicare carrier newsletters. Read them and pass them on to staff. They are critical to every practice. Keep originals in a binder within easy reach.
- CMS-1500 Claim Form Instructions (can be obtained from your Medicare carrier).
- Correct Coding Initiative (CCI) Bundling Edits. Edits can be viewed and downloaded from the CMS website at www.cms.hhs.gov.
- *The Messenger* newsletter published by Rose & Associates—available by annual subscription
- Ophthalmic Reimbursement Manual (ORM)—published by the American Society of Ophthalmic Administrators (ASOA)
- Medical dictionary such as *Stedman's* or *Dorland's*. Your technical staff will love you for it.
- *Dictionary of Eye Terminology*, 4th edition, published by Triad Publishing Company. Can be found in any major scientific bookstore.

Appendix Two

Suggested Practice Reimbursement Management Approach

Managing Reimbursment Perfomance Key Issues

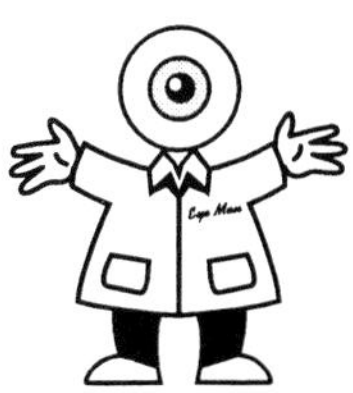

Suggested Practice
Reimbursement Management Approach

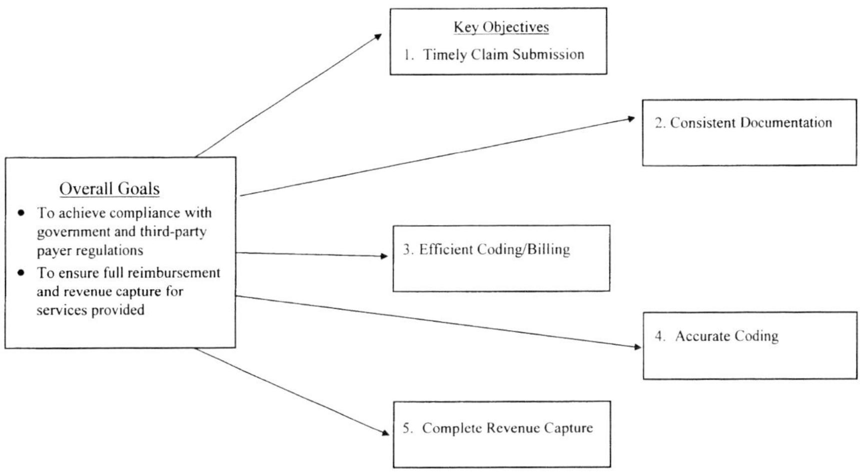

ROSE & ASSOCIATES • 402 W WHEATLAND • SUITE 150 • DUNCANVILLE, TEXAS 75116 • (972) 296-8977 • (972) 780-8546 - FAX

Managing Reimbursement Performance Key Issues

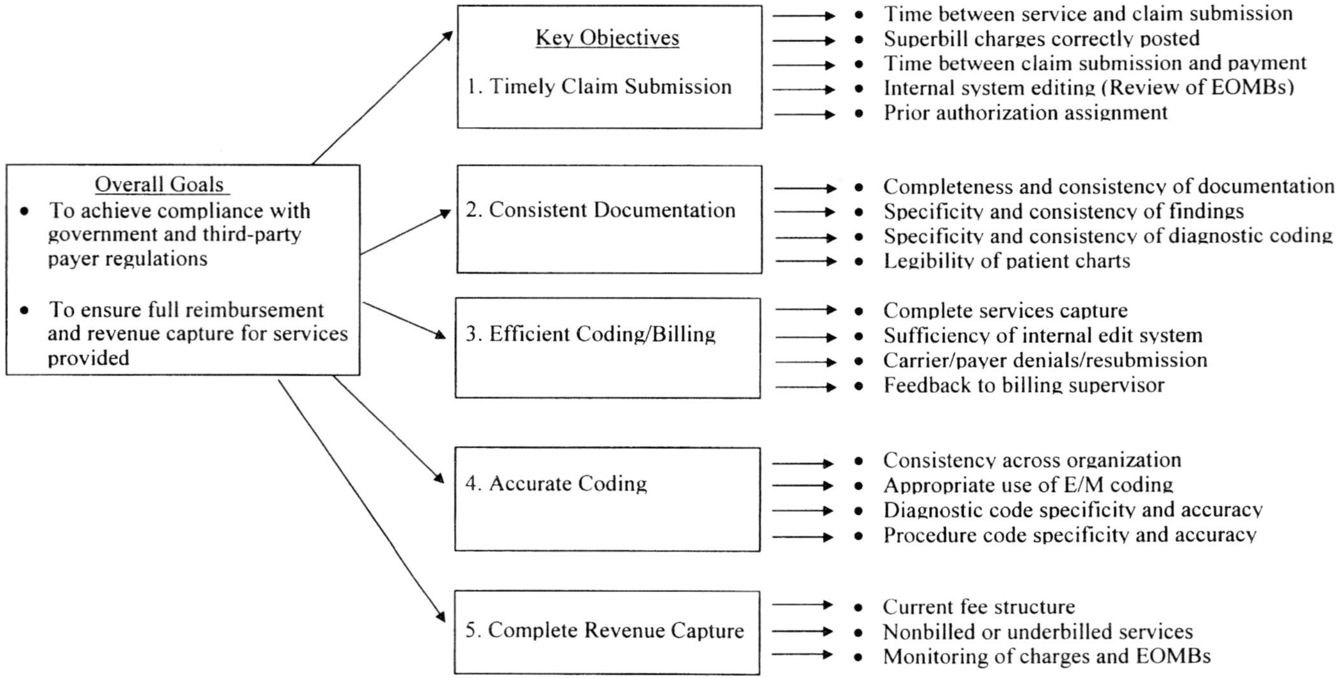

Appendix Three

Assignment of Medicare Benefits

Waiver of Payment Due to Economic Hardship

Waiver of Liability for Deluxe Frames

Advance Beneficiary Notice (ABN)

Internal Audit Worksheet

Health Insurance Claim Form

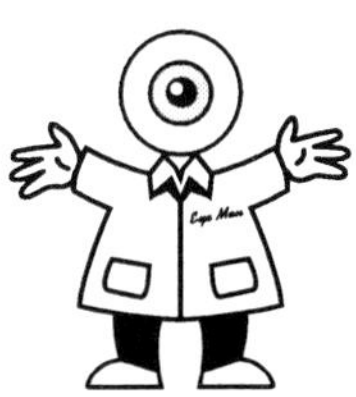

(This can be printed on letterhead or plain paper and should be a permanent part of the patient's record.)

ASSIGNMENT OF MEDICARE BENEFITS

PATIENT NAME: ______________________________

MEDICARE BENEFICIARY#: ______________________________

I request that payment of authorized Medicare benefits be made on my behalf to

______ *(Doctor' s Name / Practice Name / ASC-if applicable)* ______

for any service furnished to me by a physician of the group. I authorize any holder of medical information about me to release to the Centers for Medicare & Medicaid Services and its agents any information needed to determine these benefits payable to related services. In Medicare assigned cases, the provider agrees to accept the charge determination for the Medicare carrier and I am responsible for the Medicare deductible, co-insurance or the 20% Medicare does not pay, and for any non-covered services.

My signature below further verifies that I have not joined an HMO or other entity in which my Medicare benefits have been relinquished.

SIGNATURE: ______________________________

DATE: ______________________________

MEDIGAP OR OTHER SECONDARY INSURANCE

I request that the payment of authorized Medigap benefits be made either by me or on my behalf to *(Doctor's Name / Practice Name / ASC-if applicable)*, or any physician of that group, for services provided to me by a physician of the group. I authorize any holder of medical information about me to release it to my Medigap insurer, *(Medigap Insurer's Name)*, or any information needed to determine these benefits payable for related services.

This assignment shall remain in effect until revoked by me in writing. A photocopy of this assignment is considered as valid as the original.

SIGNATURE: ______________________________

DATE: ______________________________

(Should be Typed on Your Letterhead)

WAIVER OF PAYMENT
DUE TO ECONOMIC HARDSHIP

(Print or Type)

PATIENT NAME ______________________________

I.D. NUMBER ______________________________

STREET ADDRESS ______________________________

PHONE ______________________________

CITY ____________________ **STATE** __________ **ZIP** __________

For the reasons checked below, I am unable to pay the unreimbursed medical charges due to economic hardship. In addition, I do not have a guardian or other responsible party who can assist me with these expenses.

Please explain: *(Select all that apply)*

❑ Unemployed ❑ No insurance ❑ Bankrupt

❑ Dependent on family for support ❑ Low or fixed income

❑ Student ❑ High medical expenses

❑ Not covered by state or local welfare program

❑ Other: ______________________________

____

____

SUPPLEMENTAL INSURANCE *(If Applicable)*

COMPANY NAME ____________________ I.D# ____________________

PATIENT SIGNATURE ____________________ DATE ____________________

****

I waive the collection of unreimbursed medical charges on the above mentioned patient/family.

AUTHORIZED SIGNATURE ____________________ DATE ____________________

(Should be Typed on Your Letterhead)

WAIVER OF LIABILITY FOR DELUXE FRAMES

(Print or Type)

PATIENT'S NAME: ______________________________ **HIC#:** _______________

Having been informed that an extra charge is being made for Deluxe Frames, that this extra charge is not covered by Medicare, and that Standard Frames are available for purchase at no extra charge, I have chosen to purchase the Deluxe Frames.

PATIENT SIGNATURE ___________________________ **DATE** _______________

PRACTICE NAME
ADDRESS
TELEPHONE #

Patient's Name: ______________________ Medicare # ______________________

ADVANCE BENEFICIARY NOTICE (ABN)

NOTE: You need to make a choice about receiving these health care items or services.

We expect that Medicare will not pay for the item(s) or service(s) that are described below. Medicare does not pay for all of your health care costs. Medicare only pays for covered items and services when Medicare rules are met. The fact that Medicare may not pay for a particular item or service does not mean that you should not receive it. There may be a good reason your doctor recommended it. Right now, in your case, **Medicare probably will not pay for —**

Items or Services:
Because:

The purpose of this form is to help you make an informed choice about whether or not you want to receive these items or services, knowing that you might have to pay for them yourself. Before you make a decision about your options, you should read this entire notice carefully. Ask us to explain, if you don't understand why Medicare probably won't pay. Ask us how much these items or services will cost you **(Estimated Cost: $____________),** in case you have to pay for them yourself or through other insurance.

PLEASE CHOOSE **ONE** OPTION. CHECK **ONE** BOX. **SIGN & DATE** YOUR CHOICE.

❑ **Option 1. YES. I want to receive these items or services.**
I understand that Medicare will not decide whether to pay unless I receive these items or services. Please submit my claim to Medicare. I understand that you may bill me for items or services and that I may have to pay the bill while Medicare is making its decision. If Medicare does pay, you will refund to me any payments I made to you that are due to me. If Medicare denies payment, I agree to be personally and fully responsible for payment. That is, I will pay personally, either out of pocket or through any other insurance that I have. I understand I can appeal Medicare's decision.

❑ **Option 2. NO. I have decided not to receive these items or services.**
I will not receive these items or services. I understand that you will not be able to submit a claim to Medicare and that I will not be able to appeal your opinion that Medicare won't pay.

____

Date **(Signature of patient or person acting on patient's behalf)**

NOTE: Your health information will be kept confidential. Any information that we collect about you on this form will be kept confidential in our offices. If a claim is submitted to Medicare, your health information may be shared with Medicare. Your health information, which Medicare sees, will be kept confidential by Medicare.

OMB Approval No. 0938-0566 Form No. CMS-R-131-G

INTERNAL AUDIT WORKSHEET

DOCTOR: ____________________

SUBJECTIVE ENTRY	**YES**	**NO**
Patient's name & date of visit entered?	❑	❑
If referral, is request for consultation clearly noted?	❑	❑
Chief complaint/symptoms/reason for care noted?	❑	❑
Medical history noted?	❑	❑
Lifestyle impairment documented for cataract/YAG patient?	❑	❑
OBJECTIVE ENTRY		
Findings of exam noted?	❑	❑
Is the number of elements documented for level of service billed?	❑	❑
Is there an order for any special diagnostic tests performed?	❑	❑
Are the test results in the chart?	❑	❑
Is there an interpretation and report for each test?	❑	❑
ASSESSMENT/FINDINGS/IMPRESSIONS		
Is the final diagnosis/provisional diagnosis/suspected diagnosis noted?	❑	❑
Is patient's progress and the results of treatment noted?	❑	❑
Is there a conclusion or resolution of findings noted?	❑	❑
PLAN		
Treatment planned?	❑	❑
Any notation of management options considered but not chosen?	❑	❑
Notation of medications prescribed with dosage and regimen?	❑	❑
Referral recommended and reason for referral noted?	❑	❑
Patient education noted?	❑	❑
Patient to return for further treatment noted?	❑	❑
SPECIAL DOCUMENTATION		
Is chart signed by the physician?	❑	❑
Are chart entries legible and in ink?	❑	❑
Is a Beneficiary Signature/Medigap Signature Statement in file?	❑	❑
Is a Waiver of Liability statement signed, where applicable?	❑	❑
If consultation, is there a report of findings documented?	❑	❑
For outside referral, was a letter of findings sent to the referring doctor?	❑	❑
If surgery performed, is there an Operative Report?	❑	❑
Is a Transfer of Care agreement signed?	❑	❑
Was a copy of the Transfer of Care agreement sent to the co-manager?	❑	❑

PLEASE
DO NOT
STAPLE
IN THIS
AREA

CARRIER

PICA

HEALTH INSURANCE CLAIM FORM

PICA

1. MEDICARE (Medicare #) MEDICAID (Medicaid #) CHAMPUS (Sponsor's SSN) CHAMPVA (VA File #) GROUP HEALTH PLAN (SSN or ID) FECA BLK LUNG (SSN) OTHER (ID)

1a. INSURED'S I.D. NUMBER (FOR PROGRAM IN ITEM 1)

2. PATIENT'S NAME (Last Name, First Name, Middle Initial)

3. PATIENT'S BIRTH DATE MM DD YY SEX M F

4. INSURED'S NAME (Last Name, First Name, Middle Initial)

5. PATIENT'S ADDRESS (No., Street)

6. PATIENT RELATIONSHIP TO INSURED Self Spouse Child Other

7. INSURED'S ADDRESS (No., Street)

CITY STATE

8. PATIENT STATUS Single Married Other

CITY STATE

ZIP CODE TELEPHONE (Include Area Code) ( )

Employed Full-Time Student Part-Time Student

ZIP CODE TELEPHONE (INCLUDE AREA CODE) ( )

9. OTHER INSURED'S NAME (Last Name, First Name, Middle Initial)

10. IS PATIENT'S CONDITION RELATED TO:

11. INSURED'S POLICY GROUP OR FECA NUMBER

a. OTHER INSURED'S POLICY OR GROUP NUMBER

a. EMPLOYMENT? (CURRENT OR PREVIOUS) YES NO

a. INSURED'S DATE OF BIRTH MM DD YY SEX M F

b. OTHER INSURED'S DATE OF BIRTH MM DD YY SEX M F

b. AUTO ACCIDENT? PLACE (State) YES NO

b. EMPLOYER'S NAME OR SCHOOL NAME

c. EMPLOYER'S NAME OR SCHOOL NAME

c. OTHER ACCIDENT? YES NO

c. INSURANCE PLAN NAME OR PROGRAM NAME

d. INSURANCE PLAN NAME OR PROGRAM NAME

10d. RESERVED FOR LOCAL USE

d. IS THERE ANOTHER HEALTH BENEFIT PLAN? YES NO *If yes*, return to and complete item 9 a-d.

READ BACK OF FORM BEFORE COMPLETING & SIGNING THIS FORM.

12. PATIENT'S OR AUTHORIZED PERSON'S SIGNATURE I authorize the release of any medical or other information necessary to process this claim. I also request payment of government benefits either to myself or to the party who accepts assignment below.

SIGNED __________ DATE __________

13. INSURED'S OR AUTHORIZED PERSON'S SIGNATURE I authorize payment of medical benefits to the undersigned physician or supplier for services described below.

SIGNED __________

PATIENT AND INSURED INFORMATION

14. DATE OF CURRENT: MM DD YY ILLNESS (First symptom) OR INJURY (Accident) OR PREGNANCY(LMP)

15. IF PATIENT HAS HAD SAME OR SIMILAR ILLNESS. GIVE FIRST DATE MM DD YY

16. DATES PATIENT UNABLE TO WORK IN CURRENT OCCUPATION FROM MM DD YY TO MM DD YY

17. NAME OF REFERRING PHYSICIAN OR OTHER SOURCE

17a. I.D. NUMBER OF REFERRING PHYSICIAN

18. HOSPITALIZATION DATES RELATED TO CURRENT SERVICES FROM MM DD YY TO MM DD YY

19. RESERVED FOR LOCAL USE

20. OUTSIDE LAB? YES NO $ CHARGES

21. DIAGNOSIS OR NATURE OF ILLNESS OR INJURY. (RELATE ITEMS 1,2,3 OR 4 TO ITEM 24E BY LINE)

1. ___ . __
2. ___ . __
3. ___ . __
4. ___ . __

22. MEDICAID RESUBMISSION CODE ORIGINAL REF. NO.

23. PRIOR AUTHORIZATION NUMBER

24. A DATE(S) OF SERVICE From MM DD YY To MM DD YY	B Place of Service	C Type of Service	D PROCEDURES, SERVICES, OR SUPPLIES (Explain Unusual Circumstances) CPT/HCPCS MODIFIER	E DIAGNOSIS CODE	F $ CHARGES	G DAYS OR UNITS	H EPSDT Family Plan	I EMG	J COB	K RESERVED FOR LOCAL USE
1										
2										
3										
4										
5										
6										

25. FEDERAL TAX I.D. NUMBER SSN EIN

26. PATIENT'S ACCOUNT NO.

27. ACCEPT ASSIGNMENT? (For govt. claims, see back) YES NO

28. TOTAL CHARGE $

29. AMOUNT PAID $

30. BALANCE DUE $

31. SIGNATURE OF PHYSICIAN OR SUPPLIER INCLUDING DEGREES OR CREDENTIALS (I certify that the statements on the reverse apply to this bill and are made a part thereof.)

SIGNED DATE

32. NAME AND ADDRESS OF FACILITY WHERE SERVICES WERE RENDERED (If other than home or office)

33. PHYSICIAN'S, SUPPLIER'S BILLING NAME, ADDRESS, ZIP CODE & PHONE #

PIN# GRP#

PHYSICIAN OR SUPPLIER INFORMATION

(APPROVED BY AMA COUNCIL ON MEDICAL SERVICE 8/88) ***PLEASE PRINT OR TYPE*** APPROVED OMB-0938-0008 FORM CMS-1500 (12-90), FORM RRB-1500, APPROVED OMB-1215-0055 FORM OWCP-1500, APPROVED OMB-0720-0001 (CHAMPUS)

BECAUSE THIS FORM IS USED BY VARIOUS GOVERNMENT AND PRIVATE HEALTH PROGRAMS, SEE SEPARATE INSTRUCTIONS ISSUED BY APPLICABLE PROGRAMS.

NOTICE: Any person who knowingly files a statement of claim containing any misrepresentation or any false, incomplete or misleading information may be guilty of a criminal act punishable under law and may be subject to civil penalties.

REFERS TO GOVERNMENT PROGRAMS ONLY

MEDICARE AND CHAMPUS PAYMENTS: A patient's signature requests that payment be made and authorizes release of any information necessary to process the claim and certifies that the information provided in Blocks 1 through 12 is true, accurate and complete. In the case of a Medicare claim, the patient's signature authorizes any entity to release to Medicare medical and nonmedical information, including employment status, and whether the person has employer group health insurance, liability, no-fault, worker's compensation or other insurance which is responsible to pay for the services for which the Medicare claim is made. See 42 CFR 411.24(a). If item 9 is completed, the patient's signature authorizes release of the information to the health plan or agency shown. In Medicare assigned or CHAMPUS participation cases, the physician agrees to accept the charge determination of the Medicare carrier or CHAMPUS fiscal intermediary as the full charge, and the patient is responsible only for the deductible, coinsurance and noncovered services. Coinsurance and the deductible are based upon the charge determination of the Medicare carrier or CHAMPUS fiscal intermediary if this is less than the charge submitted. CHAMPUS is not a health insurance program but makes payment for health benefits provided through certain affiliations with the Uniformed Services. Information on the patient's sponsor should be provided in those items captioned in "Insured"; i.e., items 1a, 4, 6, 7, 9, and 11.

BLACK LUNG AND FECA CLAIMS

The provider agrees to accept the amount paid by the Government as payment in full. See Black Lung and FECA instructions regarding required procedure and diagnosis coding systems.

SIGNATURE OF PHYSICIAN OR SUPPLIER (MEDICARE, CHAMPUS, FECA AND BLACK LUNG)

I certify that the services shown on this form were medically indicated and necessary for the health of the patient and were personally furnished by me or were furnished incident to my professional service by my employee under my immediate personal supervision, except as otherwise expressly permitted by Medicare or CHAMPUS regulations.

For services to be considered as "incident" to a physician's professional service, 1) they must be rendered under the physician's immediate personal supervision by his/her employee, 2) they must be an integral, although incidental part of a covered physician's service, 3) they must be of kinds commonly furnished in physician's offices, and 4) the services of nonphysicians must be included on the physician's bills.

For CHAMPUS claims, I further certify that I (or any employee) who rendered services am not an active duty member of the Uniformed Services or a civilian employee of the United States Government or a contract employee of the United States Government, either civilian or military (refer to 5 USC 5536). For Black-Lung claims, I further certify that the services performed were for a Black Lung-related disorder.

No Part B Medicare benefits may be paid unless this form is received as required by existing law and regulations (42 CFR 424.32).

NOTICE: Any one who misrepresents or falsifies essential information to receive payment from Federal funds requested by this form may upon conviction be subject to fine and imprisonment under applicable Federal laws.

NOTICE TO PATIENT ABOUT THE COLLECTION AND USE OF MEDICARE, CHAMPUS, FECA, AND BLACK LUNG INFORMATION
(PRIVACY ACT STATEMENT)

We are authorized by CMS, CHAMPUS and OWCP to ask you for information needed in the administration of the Medicare, CHAMPUS, FECA, and Black Lung programs. Authority to collect information is in section 205(a), 1862, 1872 and 1874 of the Social Security Act as amended, 42 CFR 411.24(a) and 424.5(a) (6), and 44 USC 3101;41 CFR 101 et seq and 10 USC 1079 and 1086; 5 USC 8101 et seq; and 30 USC 901 et seq; 38 USC 613; E.O. 9397.

The information we obtain to complete claims under these programs is used to identify you and to determine your eligibility. It is also used to decide if the services and supplies you received are covered by these programs and to insure that proper payment is made.

The information may also be given to other providers of services, carriers, intermediaries, medical review boards, health plans, and other organizations or Federal agencies, for the effective administration of Federal provisions that require other third parties payers to pay primary to Federal program, and as otherwise necessary to administer these programs. For example, it may be necessary to disclose information about the benefits you have used to a hospital or doctor. Additional disclosures are made through routine uses for information contained in systems of records.

FOR MEDICARE CLAIMS: See the notice modifying system No. 09-70-0501, titled, 'Carrier Medicare Claims Record,' published in the Federal Register, Vol. 55 No. 177, page 37549, Wed. Sept. 12, 1990, or as updated and republished.

FOR OWCP CLAIMS: Department of Labor, Privacy Act of 1974, "Republication of Notice of Systems of Records," Federal Register Vol. 55 No. 40, Wed Feb. 28, 1990, See ESA-5, ESA-6, ESA-12, ESA-13, ESA-30, or as updated and republished.

FOR CHAMPUS CLAIMS: PRINCIPLE PURPOSE(S): To evaluate eligibility for medical care provided by civilian sources and to issue payment upon establishment of eligibility and determination that the services/supplies received are authorized by law.

ROUTINE USE(S): Information from claims and related documents may be given to the Dept. of Veterans Affairs, the Dept. of Health and Human Services and/or the Dept. of Transportation consistent with their statutory administrative responsibilities under CHAMPUS/CHAMPVA; to the Dept. of Justice for representation of the Secretary of Defense in civil actions; to the Internal Revenue Service, private collection agencies, and consumer reporting agencies in connection with recoupment claims; and to Congressional Offices in response to inquiries made at the request of the person to whom a record pertains. Appropriate disclosures may be made to other federal, state, local, foreign government agencies, private business entities, and individual providers of care, on matters relating to entitlement, claims adjudication, fraud, program abuse, utilization review, quality assurance, peer review, program integrity, third-party liability, coordination of benefits, and civil and criminal litigation related to the operation of CHAMPUS.

DISCLOSURES: Voluntary; however, failure to provide information will result in delay in payment or may result in denial of claim. With the one exception discussed below, there are no penalties under these programs for refusing to supply information. However, failure to furnish information regarding the medical services rendered or the amount charged would prevent payment of claims under these programs. Failure to furnish any other information, such as name or claim number, would delay payment of the claim. Failure to provide medical information under FECA could be deemed an obstruction.

It is mandatory that you tell us if you know that another party is responsible for paying for your treatment. Section 1128B of the Social Security Act and 31 USC 3801-3812 provide penalties for withholding this information.

You should be aware that P.L. 100-503, the "Computer Matching and Privacy Protection Act of 1988", permits the government to verify information by way of computer matches.

MEDICAID PAYMENTS (PROVIDER CERTIFICATION)

I hereby agree to keep such records as are necessary to disclose fully the extent of services provided to individuals under the State's Title XIX plan and to furnish information regarding any payments claimed for providing such services as the State Agency or Dept. of Health and Humans Services may request.

I further agree to accept, as payment in full, the amount paid by the Medicaid program for those claims submitted for payment under that program, with the exception of authorized deductible, coinsurance, co-payment or similar cost-sharing charge.

SIGNATURE OF PHYSICIAN (OR SUPPLIER): I certify that the services listed above were medically indicated and necessary to the health of this patient and were personally furnished by me or my employee under my personal direction.

NOTICE: This is to certify that the foregoing information is true, accurate and complete. I understand that payment and satisfaction of this claim will be from Federal and State funds, and that any false claims, statements, or documents, or concealment of a material fact, may be prosecuted under applicable Federal or State laws.

According to the Paperwork Reduction Act of 1995, no persons are required to respond to a collection of information unless it displays a valid OMB control number. The valid OMB control number for this information collection is 0938-0008. The time required to complete this information collection is estimated to average 10 minutes per response, including the time to review instructions, search existing data resources, gather the data needed, and complete and review the information collection. If you have any comments concerning the accuracy of the time estimate(s) or suggestions for improving this form, please write to: CMS, N2-14-26, 7500 Security Boulevard, Baltimore, Maryland 21244-1850.

Contributors' Biographies

Laurie K. Brown, COMT, COE, is practice administrator and **Belinda Baldwin** is business office manager for Drs. Fine, Hoffman & Packer, LLC in Eugene, Oregon. They have a combined total of 28 years of medical practice experience. Recently their practice was awarded the William E. Rose, Jr. Pinnacle Award, given by the American Society of Ophthalmic Administrators, recognizing excellence in developing and implementing exemplary polices and guidelines to help protect against erroneous or fraudulent billing practices and maintain compliance with government regulations. Laurie currently serves on the National Board of Certified Ophthalmic Executives. They can be reached at 541-687-2110.

Beth Hurley, RN, BSN, CRNO, COE, has been involved with all levels of outpatient surgery for the past 24 years. For the past five years, she has been an independent consultant providing business development and management services for new and existing facilities. She is the author of numerous articles regarding ophthalmic surgery center management and development. Having been the Director of Nurses and Administrator for multiple ophthalmic surgery centers for 14 years, she has a clear understanding of the business and operational challenges faced by free-standing ophthalmic ASCs. As a member of ASORN, she has served on the national educational committee, achieved her CRNO, and was presented the National 1999 award for Excellence in Ophthalmic Registered Nursing. She is a member of AORN and has completed the AORN Ambulatory Surgery Center Administrator Certificate Program. A member of ASOA, she attained her COE and was co-editor of the ASC edition of *Administrative Eyecare* in 2004. Since 2003, she has served as a Board member for the Outpatient Ophthalmic Surgery Society, Inc. Beth is currently Director of Clinical Development for Sovereign Healthcare, Inc., Newport Beach, California. She can be contacted at 602-432-4661 or by e-mail at bhurley@sovereignhealthcare.net or by direct e-mail at hurleybeth@aol.com.

Elizabeth Cottle, CPC, is associate administrator of the Casey Eye Institute at Oregon Health & Science University, responsible for department compliance activities. She is AAPC certified and "Specialty Proficient" in ophthalmology. Elizabeth and her practice were winners of the American Society of Ophthalmic Administrators' first annual "William E. Rose Jr. Pinnacle Award," for excellence in coding and compliance, she has over 25 years healthcare experience, with 14 years in ophthalmology. She can be reached at 503-494-6107.

Heather B. Freeland is Director of Coding and Compliance for Rose & Associates and has over 25 years experience in the health care industry. Heather served as a Medicare fair hearing officer for eight years prior to joining Rose & Associates. After graduating from the University of Miami in 1970 with a degree in biology, she began her professional career with Blue Cross and Blue Shield of Texas in the Medicare division. She worked in the reimbursement department, quality assurance auditing and post-payment medical review. She also answered congressional inquiries from federal legislators.

Heather is very familiar with Medicare legislation, regulations and instructions from the Centers for Medicare & Medicaid Services (formerly HCFA.) Her knowledge and experience enable her to answer any questions about Medicare compliance and reimbursement. She is available to conduct on-site and off-site chart audits, assist clients with responses to audit requests, prepare and handle fair hearings and administrative law judge hearings. She also serves as guest speaker at national ophthalmology meetings and conducts seminars for individual ophthalmology practices across the country.

Heather currently authors the reimbursement section of "In Your Practice," a regular department of the American Society of Ophthalmic Administrators' (ASOA) *Administrative Eyecare* magazine, and contributes regularly to *EyeWorld*, *Ophthalmology Management*, *Reimbursement and Coding Alert* and *Ocular Surgery News*. Heather can be reached at 1-800-720-9667 or emailed at results@roseandassociates.com.

Richard Gable has more than 20 years of experience in the healthcare industry. Rick is considered a leading authority on managed care, marketing and practice management. He is one of the nation's foremost expert's in developing profitable medical/surgery, ambulatory surgery center, routine eye and eyewear capitation arrangements. He can be reached at 949-609-0149 or DHC38@aol.com.

Stephen W. Gilkeson has served as the Executive Administrator for the Young Eye Institute in Lawton, Oklahoma since 1988. Specializing in cataract removal with lens implant, YEI has grown to represent one of the largest full-service eye care facilities in Oklahoma and North Central Texas. The Young Eye Institute was one of the first winners of the William E. Rose, Jr. Pinnacle Awards. He can be reached at 580-353-5860.

Alan E. Reider's practice is limited to health law. He represents physicians, suppliers, hospitals, laboratories, as well as national health care corporations. This representation focuses on regulatory issues involving Federal programs, as well as relationships with third party payors, counseling in the area of fraud and abuse, principally the Federal anti-kickback and Stark self-referral laws as well as state restrictions, development of compliance programs and defending providers and practitioners in False Claims Act, Civil Money Penalty, and suspension and exclusion actions.

Mr. Reider has extensive experience working with ophthalmology practices. He serves as outside counsel to the Society for Excellence in Eyecare as well as the International Society for Refractive Surgery. He is the author of the Model Compliance Program for Ophthalmologists, published by the American Society of Ophthalmic Administrators. Mr. Reider serves as the Regulatory and Legislative Section Editor for *Ocular Surgery News*. He can be reached at 202-857-6462.

List of Acronyms/Glossary

List of Acronyms

ABN – Advance Benefit Notice
AK – Astigmatic keratotomy
ALJ – Administrative Law Judge
AMA – American Medical Association
A/R – Accounts Receivable
ASC – Ambulatory Surgical Center
AORN – Association of Operating Room Nurses
CCI – Correct Coding Initiative
CMS – Centers for Medicare and Medicaid Services
DME – Durable Medical Equipment
DO – Doctor of Osteopathy
DON – Director of Nursing
E & M – Evaluation and Management
EMC – Electronic Media Claim
FTE – Full Time Employee
HCPCS – Health Care Financing Administration Common Procedure Coding System
HIPAA – Health Insurance Portability Accountability Act
HMO – Health Maintenance Organization
IBNR – Incurred but not reported
IPA – Independent Practice Association
LASIK – Laser in situ keratomileusis
OCR – Optical Character Recognition
OIG – Office of the Inspector General

Glossary

Actual Charge – The physician's billed or submitted charge, which is the amount Medicare will pay if it is lower than the Medicare payment schedule amount.

Ambulatory Surgical Center (ASC): A facility (either freestanding or affiliated with a hospital) operated exclusively to provide outpatient surgical services to patients through an agreement with the Centers for Medicare and Medicaid Services.

Balance Bill: A physician's charge exceeding the Medicare-allowed charge.

Beneficiary: A person eligible for benefits under an insurance plan. Under Part B of Medicare, Americans over 65, many disabled individuals, and certain individuals with end-stage renal disease can become beneficiaries by paying a monthly premium.

Bundling: The use of a single payment for a group of related services.

Carrier (Medicare): A private contractor that administers claims processing and payment for Part B services.

Centers for Medicare and Medicaid Services (CMS): Agency within the U.S. Department of Health and Human Services that administers the Medicare program.

Clean Claim: A claim that has not been rejected for additional information.

Coding: A mechanism for identifying and describing physician's services for purposes of submitting claims for payment.

Copayment: A fixed dollar amount per service that is the responsibility of the beneficiary.

Deductible: The annual amount that Medicare beneficiaries must meet before Medicare will begin paying for service in any years.

Department of Health and Human Services (HHS): Department within the U.S. Government that is responsible for administering health and social welfare programs.

Fee for Service: A system of paying physicians for individual medical services rendered, as opposed to paying them salaries or capitation payments. The Medicare Fee Schedule is an example of a service payment system.

Fee Schedule: A list of predetermined payments for units of medical service.

Global Service: A package of clinically related services treated as a unit for purposes of billing, coding, or payment.

Health Maintenance Organization (HMO): A prepaid, organized health care plan. Individuals are enrolled in the plan, and services are provided through a system of affiliated providers. Comprehensive benefits are financed by prepaid premiums with limited copayments.

Intraocular Lens (IOL): An artificial lens that may be implanted to replace the natural lens after cataract surgery.

Limiting Charge: The maximum amount that a nonparticipating physician is permitted to charge for a service; a limit on balance billing.

Medicaid: A joint federal-state program of federal matching grants to the states to provide health insurance for categories of poor and medically indigent. States determine eligibility, payments, and benefits consistent with federal standards.

Medicare Fee Schedule (MFS): The resource-based fee schedule currently used by Medicare to pay for physician's services.

Part A (Medicare): The hospital insurance program, which covers the cost of hospital and related post-hospital services. Eligibility is normally based on prior payment of payroll taxes. Beneficiaries are responsible for an initial deductible per spell of illness and copayments for some services.

Part B (Medicare) The Supplementary Medical Insurance program, which covers the cost of physician services, outpatient laboratory and X-ray tests, durable medical equipment, outpatient hospital care, and certain other services. Part B requires payment of a monthly premium, which covers roughly 25% of program costs. Beneficiaries are responsible for a deductible and coinsurance payment for most covered services.

Part C (Medicare) The "Medicare + Choice" program through which an organization can contract with the Centers for Medicare and Medicaid Services (CMS) Health Care Financing Administration to offer a variety of managed care programs.

Peer Review Organization (PRO). An organization contracting with CMS to review the medical necessity and the quality of care provided to Medicare beneficiaries; Utilization and Quality Control Peer Review Organization.

Practice Expense: The cost of nonphysician resources incurred by the physician to provide services. Examples are salaries and fringe benefits received by nurses, physician assistants, and receptionists who are employed by the physician.

Premium: An amount paid periodically by program beneficiaries to purchase medical insurance benefits. Medicare premiums are updated on an annual basis.

Prospective Payment System (PPS): The Medicare system used to pay hospitals for inpatient hospital services; based on the DRG classification system.

Submitted Charge: The actual charge submitted to the patient or payer.

Supplier: A provider of health care services, other than a practitioner, that is permitted to bill under Medicare Part B. Supplies include independent laboratories, durable medical equipment providers, ambulance services, prosthetists, and portable X-ray providers.

Third-Party Payer: A party or group other than the recipient of health care services which has contractually agreed to assume financial responsibility for the services, such as an insurance company or a governmental body.

Upcode: To bill more than the customary fee for a provided service.

Index

ASOA

American Society of Ophthalmic Administrators

Founded in 1986, the American Society of Ophthalmic Administrators (ASOA) is the premier organization for the *business* side of ophthalmic practice. Serving physicians, administrators, managers, and office staff, its mission is to advance the skills and professionalism of ophthalmic practice management.

As a member of ASOA you become part of a worldwide network of professionals who confront the same challenges you do in your quest to run a successful, cost-effective practice. Check us out online at www.asoa.org for the most up-to-date list of benefits.

Membership Application

Last Name: First Name: MI:

Email address

Company/Practice Name

Address

City: State: Zip:

Country:

Is this a business □ or home □ address

Is this a business □ or home □ phone

Your role: □ Physician/Administrator/Manager □ Office Staff □ Clinical Staff □ Vendor □ Consultant

Form of payment: □ VISA □ MasterCard

Account # Exp. date: ( ) Month ( ) Year

Name on card:

I authorize ASCRS/ASOA to charge this account in the amount of $250 for a 1-year membership.

Signature:

Return form to: ASOA, 4000 Legato Road, Suite 700, Fairfax, VA 22033. Fax to: 703-591-5020. Questions: 703-591-2220. (Code: PINTO)